"This book offers needed help and hope for those who have a loved one experiencing dementia. John Dunlop's training as a medical doctor, along with his understanding of what the Bible teaches us about our bodies and our souls, gives him a unique perspective from which to address this crucial issue."

Dennis Rainey, president, FamilyLife

"Finding this book is like discovering a wonderful treasure. John Dunlop has mined decades of experience as geriatrician, son of a mother with dementia, bioethics expert, and active church member to help the rest of us make sense of a condition that seems to rob people of every shred of dignity. Drawing on the glorious biblical truth of every person's creation in the image of God, Dunlop shows that dignity cannot be lost even in the face of dementia. People entering or anticipating the experience of dementia, as well as their family, friends, and caregivers—in other words, nearly everyone—will find in this book the grace they need to cope with its challenges."

John Kilner, professor of bioethics and contemporary culture, Trinity International University; author, *Why People Matter* and *Dignity and Destiny*

"Almost thirty years ago, my mother died of complications springing from nine years of Alzheimer's Disease. During those nine years I read several helpful books that described the stages of the disease, what to expect, and how to respond. Nowadays similar resources are found on the web. But there is nothing quite like John Dunlop's book on dementia. Decades of experience as a geriatrician and a devout Christian combine to help other believers think through dementia—what it means, how to trust God when you see its onset (in yourself or in friends and relatives), and, yes, how God glorifies himself and brings strength to his people precisely in the midst of such horrendous, ravaging illness. This book will help you become a better caregiver; more importantly, it will help you become a more mature and thoughtful Christian. It may even help you become a better patient."

D. A. Carson, research professor of New Testament, Trinity Evangelical Divinity School; cofounder, The Gospel Coalition

"My father-in-law resided with us through his eight-year journey with Alzheimer's. As a physician, I had taken care of patients with dementia, but then I lived with the disease. The best way to help a friend or family member dealing with this illness is to give them a copy of this book. It is an invaluable resource."

David Stevens, chief executive officer, Christian Medical & Dental Associations

"*Finding Grace in the Face of Dementia* is a remarkably helpful book on the increasingly common phenomenon of dementia. Growing out of his medical practice as a geriatric physician and his experience as a caregiver for his parents, both of whom suffered from dementia, John Dunlop writes for those who struggle with this disease, for caregivers, and for members of the body of Christ eager to lean in and love well in these difficult circumstances. This book ably and understandably covers the waterfront medically, theologically, practically, and experientially. Combining compassionate kindness, sober realism, appropriate anguish and lament, and ultimate confidence in God's love and grace, Dunlop both encourages and fortifies those who suffer and those who give care. This book rings true to my own experience with my mother, who suffered from dementia for twenty years. May this much-needed resource be used widely and mightily in the days ahead."

Steven C. Roy, associate professor of pastoral theology, Trinity Evangelical Divinity School

"Dementia may well be the most feared diagnosis in the Western world, and this book is a timely contribution to a community in need of education and encouragement. Dunlop does not gloss over the challenges that dementia can bring but takes us by the hand and leads us sympathetically through the various aspects of the illness. Dunlop's extensive experience allows him to contribute rich practical and spiritual wisdom for those walking this path. I highly recommend it as a guide."

Megan Best, palliative care practitioner; bioethicist

Finding Grace in the Face of Dementia

Finding Grace in the Face of Dementia

John Dunlop, MD

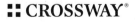

WHEATON, ILLINOIS

To those who
seek to love and care
for people with dementia
in ways that honor God

Contents

Introduction

Dementia, dignity, and honoring God—you must be kidding! Chances are you have never seen those three thoughts in the same sentence. How can such a tragedy as dementia be dignified, and how in the world can God be honored through it?

As followers of Jesus, we should desire God to be honored in all things, so that includes our approach to the tragedies of life, even dementia. A number of years ago, when I started questioning these issues, I was talking to a friend about a paper I wanted to write on how dementia can bring honor to God. I recall telling my friend that I did not know what I was going to say but that it was going to be very short. Well, the more I got into it, the more I realized there are many ways in which God can graciously use the tragedy of dementia to honor himself. That short paper has become this book.

Over and over again I have seen God honored when others respect the inherent dignity of those afflicted with dementia. It happens because the dignity of everyone, including those with dementia, is rooted in nothing less than the fact that they were made in the image of God. Dementia is common today and will become increasingly so in the future. If we are to live faithful to our Lord, Jesus Christ, we need to learn how we can respect the dignity of those who suffer from it and in the process honor God.

At the outset we must have a common understanding of dignity, since the term has a wide variety of meanings. Some define *dignity* as something intrinsic to being a person. Others think of it as an individual's reputation, while some look at it as people's ability to respect themselves and be in control of their lives. When used in connection with the end of life, many use the word *dignity* to refer to freedom from pain and dependence. None of these are what I have in mind. Scripture teaches that all human beings are made in the image of God, which makes them distinct from the rest of God's creation. Humans are loved by God to the extent that his Son died to allow those who believe in him to enjoy his presence forever. These two facts impart a dignity rooted not in who they are or in what they can accomplish but only in God himself. It is true of all persons, including those with the most severe dementia. Now, in addition to a God-given dignity common to all, there may be other sources of dignity that vary from person to person. Some may be more dignified in their character, and others acquire dignity through their accomplishments, but these sources of dignity are added to their inherent, God-given dignity.

As you read, you will notice that I never refer to those afflicted with dementia as "the demented." No! I always refer to them as "people with dementia." I never want to think of dementia as something that defines who they are. They are first and foremost people even though afflicted with the dreaded disease called "dementia."

The Good, the Bad, and the Ugly

Dementia can be experienced in a wide variety of ways. Just to illustrate, I'll share with you three stories from my direct experience. You will see that they represent the good, the bad, and the ugly.

Jessie illustrates the good. At eighty-six, she was still the life of the party. After spending decades on the mission field, she developed dementia, became progressively confused, and was no longer able to live at home with her husband. When I visited her in the nursing home, she was invariably sitting with a group of friends animatedly telling stories of her life in Congo. She would get to the punch line, slap her thigh, and laugh contagiously. Her friends, gathered around her, had a great time. Now, did it really matter that Jessie told the same three stories over and over? It didn't to her friends! They enjoyed them at the moment, even though they did not remember them. She was happy, she had a meaningful role in the lives of others, and she enjoyed talking about her Lord and the work she had seen him do. Unfortunately Jessie's story is not typical, nor is it even common, but it does show a "good" side to dementia.

The bad is seen in the experience of my mother. Mom was one of the kindest, most loving women I have ever known. She was widowed at eighty and continued to live independently in a senior-adult facility for many years. People regularly invited her to eat with them, as they loved her sweet spirit and happy demeanor. She had a real ministry to the dying and, in rotation with some other residents, would go sit with those who were dying in the nursing wing of the community and softly sing to them her favorite hymns. Slowly, however, she began to lose some of her abilities. She caused several small fires by forgetting to turn off the stove; and she would occasionally lose her way when returning to her apartment. The administration told us, her children, that it was time for her to move into the dementia section of the facility. After praying together, we met with her to discuss making a change. Though we had expected her to resist, we were thrilled when she graciously consented to the move. Over her year there, she became increasingly forgetful, confused, and at times agitated. One time she struck another resident, which was totally out of character for Mom. She was then moved to the nursing wing, where she became increasingly boisterous and at times combative. She was generally nice to us, but clearly her personality had changed. Eventually, she did not recognize us as her children, yet it seemed she knew we loved her. I feel sorry that I had to place Mom's story into the "bad" category, but she is far from unique, as most patients with dementia fall into this category at some point.

13

When I think of the "ugly," my mind goes to James. He had been the executive of his family. Raised by a domineering father, he tragically followed that example well. Married fifty years, James and his wife had three daughters. They were his pride and joy, while they, in turn, loved him dearly. But James was in charge, and he left no question about that. In his mid-seventies he became increasingly forgetful and confused. He was unable to recognize that he was failing and still insisted on being the boss. He would wake up at 3:00 a.m. and insist that his disabled wife cook him his breakfast. Not being able to do so, she would call their daughter who lived nearby. She responded dutifully and cooked his eggs to his precise order, but then he'd go into a rage because he thought he had ordered her to make French toast. She was broken to tears. Such things began happening all too frequently until eventually the family, in desperation, had to make arrangements for James at a dementia-care facility. James's case was "ugly" and, though somewhat less common, not rare.

Yes, dementia comes in all shapes and sizes. But what actually do we mean by *dementia*? At its simplest, *dementia* is a compound word. The prefix *de-* signifies "removal of," and *ment* comes from the same root as *mental*, so literally *dementia* means "less brain." The term *dementia* is falling out of vogue. Now it is more correct to refer to *major neurocognitive impairment*. Since that is a mouthful and not widely understood, I will continue to use the word *dementia*.

There is often confusion between dementia and Alzheimer's disease. Dementia is a larger category of which about 70 percent is Alzheimer's. In this book I will usually speak of dementia rather than restricting my comments to Alzheimer's. There are a number of other kinds of dementia, as well, as you will see in later chapters. I also comment that though this book focuses on the dementias typically associated with the later years of life, the principles I share are relevant to those with cognitive impairment at any stage of life, including those in their younger years who have intellectual development disorders (formerly termed "mental retardation") and those who have suffered brain injury.

The Challenges of Dementia

Our older years can have many challenges. "Old age is not for cowards," as one of my dementia patients told me at every appointment. Each time she said it, she laughed, thinking it was the first time she'd ever said it. The apostle Paul expressed it differently: "Through many tribulations we must enter the kingdom of God" (Acts 14:22). I often speak of the "four Ds" of our later years: depression, disease, dementia, and death. Any one of these can be difficult, but, for many, dementia is the greatest challenge. It can be a massive tragedy not only for the patient but, perhaps even more, for those who love and care for them. Dementia can progress over as many as twenty years before it finally leads to death, and even then it can leave horrible memories for the survivors. It is further tragic, as we will see, for while there are many ways to improve the quality of the life of those with dementia, there are currently no cures.

It bothers me how many people fear getting dementia, even more than they fear cancer or death. This fear comes from at least two reasons. First, many have had bad experiences with dementia sufferers, and they don't want to succumb themselves. Second, and on a more fundamental level, dementia is a threat to the basic values of Western culture. Society values youth, wit, independence, and control. We are tempted to equate our individual value with our IQs and our ability to accomplish things. Dementia will likely threaten both. One lesson we can learn from those with dementia is that value can be found in something other than our cognitive abilities and usefulness. As we progress through this book, we will see that there is great value in the fact that people with dementia can still experience feelings and are capable of relationships. Of even greater value is the fact that they, being made in the image of God and loved by him, possess inherent dignity. The experience of dementia can help teach us what our true value is, and embracing it may make the prospect of dementia less threatening and fearful.

Finally, dementia is a challenge because it is so common and will become more so. At the time of my writing, there are over six million Americans who suffer from dementia. Roughly speaking, 5 percent of Americans have dementia at age sixty-five, and this number will double roughly every seven years. Doing the math tells us that by age ninety, nearly half will have some form of dementia. Fortunately, the rate of increase begins to slow down by that stage of life. These numbers mean that one-third of seniors will die with some form of the disease, but not necessarily from it. In part this is the consequence of the wonderful life-prolonging technologies and healthier lifestyles we now have. It is certainly a bad result for a good reason. Dementia has a significant economic impact. Estimates are that the total cost of dementia to this country is approximately 220 billion dollars a year. That number is staggering, as it is almost half the total amount spent on public education. Dementia will become more and more of a problem for society as a whole but also for the church of Jesus Christ, which will need to assume a greater role in the care of those who suffer from it.

My Interest in Dementia

This book flows out of many of my own passions. First is my trust in God and love for him and his Word, the Bible. There I learn that God is good, loving, and all-powerful. The difficult challenges of life do not come by accident. No! Our sovereign God brings them into our lives with purpose. Over the years as I have been confronted with dementia, I have failed to recognize any purpose for it, yet I believe it is my responsibility to search out what God's reason may be. This book is my attempt to explore God's possible purposes in allowing this horrible disease. But even when I do not fully understand, I have learned I can still trust him. My trust in God is not ultimately rooted in how well my life is going or how comfortable and happy I am. God has already proven his love for me by coming into this evil world in the person of Jesus, dying on the cross, and demonstrating his power over life and death by rising from the dead. Surely a God who loved me to that extent can be trusted even through the challenges of dementia, whether I understand its purpose or not.

Second, I enjoy both the science of medicine as well as the wonderful relationships I have had throughout my career as a geriatrician. Helping patients who suffer from dementia and their families has been a large part of that practice. The work isn't always joyful, because I regularly observe their frustration and anger. I have tried my best to keep up with the findings of dementia research and apply that knowledge to my treatment of patients, including prescribing the newest medicines, even though I am frustrated with how little benefit they have. Many think that apart from these medications, little can be done to lessen the suffering. Yet this is not true. I, along with other professionals, have come to realize that there is something more important than dispensing medications to deal with dementia, and that is treating its victims with respect and dignity. For that reason, one of my goals is to help caretakers know how to honor God as they relate to the afflicted.

The third reason is personal. I have a strong genetic predisposition to dementia and may well be its victim someday. Recently I have joked with my friends, saying that I want to get this book written soon before it becomes an autobiography.

Is There a Christian Approach to Dementia?

Jesus set us a wonderful example of how to truly love others. In addition, the Bible contains many helpful principles for dementia care. Does this mean that there is a distinctively Christian approach to dealing with dementia? Most certainly not! But there are right ways, and there are wrong ways. I find it remarkable how frequently the right way is consistent with traditional Judeo-Christian values as revealed in the Scriptures and illustrated by

Jesus. I know wonderful caregivers, both professionals and laypersons, who are doing an awesome job yet have little knowledge of Jesus. Most experts in the field who give profoundly sage advice do not claim to be Christian or provide any biblical basis for their approach.

Even though there may not always be a significant difference between the approaches of Christian and non-Christian caregivers, there may be a huge difference in why they follow those approaches and in the resources they have to draw on to do it well. Distinctively Christian care should spring from an unselfish love for those in need, not from a sense of obligation or the desire to receive recognition. One of my frequent prayers is that I will serve my patients out of the fullness that comes from knowing how much God loves me and has given to me. I dread the thought of trying to please people so that I can feel good about myself or receive appreciation and praise.

Christians also have unique resources to help them, including the wisdom and love of God that comes through the indwelling presence of the Holy Spirit, the ability to pray for God's comfort and help, and a church body willing to pitch in and assist. Perhaps above all else, caregivers who rely on God can appreciate the fact that they, too, have a caregiver in heaven, the Lord Jesus.

About *Finding Grace in the Face of Dementia*

In thinking about how God can be honored in and even through dementia, several key questions arise, and the answers to those are intertwined through this book. These include:

- Do we view people with dementia as whole persons, or does their personhood diminish with their cognitive ability?
- How can a good and powerful God allow such a tragedy? Is dementia meaningless, and if not, what are God's purposes?
- What is it like to experience dementia?

- What strategies can allow us to honor God as we navigate the challenges of dementia?

Throughout the book I will be sharing stories largely taken from my personal experience (though all the names have been changed). Throughout is woven the story of one couple I know well, whom I call Dave and Denise, although I have modified several aspects of their experience to better illustrate my points. As you will see, they have found grace to deal with dementia in a way that honors God.

The approach I start with is to view dementia in the context of the storyline of the Bible—creation, fall, redemption, and future hope. Then I develop some background information to allow us to understand what it must be like to experience dementia. The next part of the book is dedicated to those who care for people with dementia. We need to understand that while the job is really tough, it is associated with certain rewards. The book will conclude with an explanation of a number of ways in which God can be honored through dementia.

My purpose in writing this book is to provide a theological lens through which we can view dementia and then give a number of practical ways in which it can be applied. I trust it will be useful for those who are developing the disease as well as those who care for people at any stage of it. I also hope that many professional caregivers, whether doctors, nurses, chaplains, or social workers, will benefit from this read. In addition, I believe it will be useful for pastors, other church leaders, and members of ethics committees. I suspect that most readers will be followers of Jesus, but I truly hope that the book will be read by non-Christians as well. I am impressed by how many who do not embrace the Christian faith nevertheless hold the life and teachings of Jesus in high regard. My desire is that they will profit from a deeper consideration of how Jesus would respond to dementia.

I have chosen to conclude each chapter with a prayer. I encourage you to pray along with me, for I am fully aware that without God's speaking to you through this book, my time to write it and your time reading it will be wasted. It is also true, when we face tragedies such as dementia, that we do not always know what to pray for. I offer my prayers as one potential model, but fundamentally it will be the Holy Spirit who will lead you to pray aright.

So now let's launch into this very challenging discussion.

Prayer

Dear Father, I need to know more about dementia. It is all too common and all too devastating. I am intrigued with the thought that you may actually have some purpose in this terrible disease. As I think further about this, my prayer is that you, by your Holy Spirit working through your Word, will be my teacher. I pray that you will be honored both in my own spirit and in others as I relate to them. I pray this for my good and for your honor. Amen.

1

God and Dementia

I hate dementia. When I saw it developing in both of my parents, it was hard to see these beautiful, loving people incapacitated by the changes in their minds, even though their dementias were not the worst cases I have known—not by far. But even while I lament this tragedy, I am still totally convinced that God is both good and strong and that dementia was in his plan for them. One of my favorite psalms puts it like this: "Once God has spoken; twice have I heard this: that power belongs to God, and that to you, O Lord, belongs steadfast love" (Ps. 62:11–12).

In his love God was able to prevent their dementias but chose not to. How am I to respond? Is he really not as good or loving as I had thought? Is he not strong enough to control dementia? I know these are valid questions to ponder; perhaps you are asking them yourself. When I confront such challenges, I have learned that I have to go back to the very basics of my faith and begin to see my struggles in the full light of Scripture. Granted, we will not find in the Bible any mention of dementia, but we do find some enduring principles that help us understand this disease and allow us to respond to it in God-honoring ways.

God Has Purpose in All Things

One of those principles is that God has a purpose in all that happens. He never makes mistakes. As we face dementia in ourselves or loved ones, we can identify with the psalmist who wrote, "I cry out to God Most High, to God who fulfills his purpose for me" (Ps. 57:2). Even while recognizing that God had a purpose in what he did, the psalmist still cried out to God in his need. The more we get to know God, the more we can trust him, even when we may not understand why he does what he does. I love what Paul says: "Oh, the depth of the riches and wisdom and knowledge of God! How unsearchable are his judgments and how inscrutable his ways!" (Rom. 11:33). Once we recognize that in his infinite wisdom he has a purpose in dementia, there is no problem affirming his love and power.

Life Is Not about Us but about God

The second underlying principle we must take from Scripture is that fundamentally our lives are not all about us but about God. "In the beginning, God . . ." (Gen. 1:1). That is where we have to start. Before anything else, God was there. He alone exists simply because he exists. He was primary; everything else was secondary. He was Creator; everything else was created. He introduced himself to Moses as "I AM" (Ex. 3:14). He gave no explanation but in a sense simply said, "Here I am—just accept me." The apostle Paul expressed it clearly: "For from him and through him and to him are all things. To him be glory forever. Amen" (Rom. 11:36). Our universe came from him, it is daily sustained by him, and its ultimate purpose will be fulfilled in his being glorified.

This means our lives should focus on God. One of the challenges is that he allows us to enjoy so much in this life that it is easy to think that our reason for existence is to live comfortably and find happiness in every way we can. We must never discount the many blessings God pours into our earthly lives and be grateful for them. But when we focus only on the gifts and not on the giver, we are grievously wrong. Life is fundamentally about coming to know him personally and finding fulfillment and joy in nothing other than God himself. He alone can satisfy our deepest longings. If we are settling for the pleasure we get only in ourselves and in this world, we are accepting something second-rate. Adopting this God-centered view of life is critical to rightly viewing dementia. It is not simply about dementia disrupting our comfort and happiness; this disease becomes a tool that God uses to accomplish his ultimate purpose: his honor, his glory.

Dementia Was Not Part of God's Good Creation

Seven times in Genesis 1 we are told that the world God made was good, meaning it conformed perfectly to God's character. It was filled with love, beauty, joy, righteousness, and satisfying work for our first parents. There was no human death, no disease, no pain or suffering. Most important, for our present purposes, there was no dementia.

All Humans Are Made in God's Image and Are His by Right of Creation

The high point of God's creation was humans. He created us, and so by right we all belong to him. The psalmist caught the significance of this when he wrote, "The earth is the LORD's and the fullness thereof, the world and those who dwell therein" (Ps. 24:1). Applying this truth to dementia victims means that they, too, belong to God just as much as anyone else, and we must treat them accordingly.

God made all of us with both minds and bodies, and who we are is an essential unity of these; both are equally important to our identity. There is no such thing as a half person. We cannot afford to discredit the importance of our physical bodies and emphasize our minds or do the opposite. Our bodies may get sick and not function well, but we are still persons. Our minds may get sick and not function well, but we are still persons. We will see that dementia may devastate some of our brain's abilities, such as memory and rationality, but we still have feelings and are able to enjoy human relationships. We are still whole persons who belong to God.

That each of us is God's creation and belongs to him is reason enough to treat everyone with respect. But there is an even more significant basis for doing so: each of us has been made in the image and likeness of God.[1] That we are made in God's image is the first thing God declared about humankind and so distinguished us from all the rest of creation. Scripture doesn't say we are the exact image of God but rather that we are made in, or according to, God's image. Only Jesus is the exact image of God (Col. 1:15; Heb. 1:3). Being made in God's image conveys a special dignity to all men and women, and this dignity does not depend on how closely our character resembles God, how smart we are, or what wonderful things we do. The fact of human dignity is equally as true of the Nobel Laureate as of the most severe dementia sufferer who is totally dependent on others.

Sin Led to Dementia but Did Not Diminish God's Image

Our first parents were not content to live in loving relationship with their Creator and decided that merely reflecting his image was not enough for them. They wanted to be even more like God. So they disobeyed the one command God had given them. In that single act of rebellion, sin entered the human race. God's good creation began to unravel in almost every way. As a result of man's disobedience, death came alongside life, and alongside goodness came evil, alongside love came hate, and alongside health came disease, including dementia.

But even as sin disrupted so much of God's good creation, one thing it did not destroy was the image of God in all human beings. This is a key concept and worth belaboring, for it means that even those severely afflicted with dementia share equally with all of humanity in the image of God with its inherent dignity. We see this here: "Whoever sheds the blood of man, by man shall his blood be shed, for God made man in his own image" (Gen. 9:6). After the flagrant sin that led to the flood, God placed a special protection on mankind because they were "in his own image."

We get another fascinating glimpse from the New Testament, where James writes, concerning our tongues, "With it we bless our Lord and Father, and with it we curse people who are made in the likeness [image] of God" (James 3:9). Even when people are such scoundrels that we want to curse them, they still bear the image of God. Sin did not destroy the image of God nor do we get any indication in Scripture that it diminished it any more than damaging a building alters its blueprint. Martin Luther King understood the significance of this when he said, "There are no gradations in the image of God."[2]

However, sin did damage our ability to reflect the image of God, and it did so in profound ways. Further, when sin entered the world, it compromised our ability to enjoy our lives on earth. This is seen in countless ways, but one of them is dementia and the way it wreaks havoc in the lives of its sufferers and those who love and care for them. We are right to be frustrated and even angry at dementia, leading us to cry out to God, lament the tragedy, and look for God's help to respond to it rightly.

God Uses Bad to Accomplish Good

One of the striking things the Bible teaches us about God is how he takes some of the most difficult circumstances of life and transforms them for his own purposes. We see that dramatically in the case of sin itself. God's glory is certainly seen in the marvels of his beautiful creation. But we see even more of his glory in the way he dealt with sin. In spite of our turning our backs on God, he loved us to the extent that he sent his Son to suffer and die to bring us back into relationship with him. Similarly, God takes many of the most difficult challenges of life and turns them around, enabling us to appreciate how great he is. His purpose may not be our immediate comfort but our long-term ability to find our greatest joy in him. Joni Eareckson Tada, who is quadriplegic, is well known for saying of God, "Always permitting what he hates to accomplish something he loves."[3] Pastor Tim Keller explains it clearly: "The evils of life can be justified if we recognize that the world was primarily created to be a place where people find God and grow spiritually into all they were designed to be."[4] One of those things that God may hate, one of those evils of life, is dementia. Yet, as we will see, God can use dementia to allow us to know more of his goodness and to honor him.

We Will Be Like Him

God is in the process of calling out from mankind a group of people as his own. He gives them the ability to trust him by faith and makes them his children. He chooses them not according to how good they are, for no one is good enough to merit what he gives. Instead, he chooses them to show how good he is. Then he begins the slow process of restoring them fully to his image, which they were made in. Paul writes, "Those whom he foreknew he also predestined to be conformed to the image of his Son. . . . And those whom he predestined he also called, and those whom he called he also justified, and those whom he justified he also glorified" (Rom. 8:29–30). Now, here is the key point. All those he has chosen will increasingly conform to his image, and in the end all will enter into his glory.[5] This transformation is based not on their abilities or IQ but on God's choice and plan. The apostle John put it simply: "We shall be like him" (1 John 3:2).

Robert Davis, a pastor who experienced dementia, reflected on his final destiny and wrote, "How can I stand to look at this disaster [referring to his dementia] that medical science predicts will most probably overtake me? If I were not a Christian, I do not know how I could stand it. However, since I am a Christian, I can stand it by looking beyond it—looking beyond and considering the glories of heaven where each one of these things will be gone forever and be replaced by perfection, glory, and joy."[6]

As Christians we can confront dementia with confidence that God will accomplish his purpose and his glory. In that we can find joy and hope. We know in the future all believers, including those with dementia, will stand in his presence as whole people reflecting more of his image. Such is the destiny of those suffering from dementia, including the most severe forms of it. They will be completely restored as whole people, body and soul together, fully able to enjoy the richness of God through all eternity. That destiny is a further source of the dignity they possess even in the compromised state they live in today.

But in the meantime, one way we can be helped to honor God through the experience of dementia is by understanding more about it, which is what we'll consider next.

Prayer

Heavenly Father, dementia is scary. The very thought of it terrifies me. I confess it is difficult to believe you are loving and strong while at the same time you allow this tragedy. Help me believe you have a purpose in all that you do. I want to trust you, but it will be easier if I can get a glimpse of the purpose you intend through dementia. By your Spirit, guide my thinking and my emotional responses. I pray this for my good and for your honor. Amen.

2

What Should We Know
about Dementia?

Allow me to introduce you to Dave and Denise, two dear friends, whose story I will be sharing throughout this book. Both in their mid-sixties, they have had a good marriage for thirty-three years. They have three loving and supportive children. Dave is a medical technician, and Denise works in a high school cafeteria. They keep themselves in good health, eat wisely, and exercise on a regular schedule. Having been Christians for most of their adult lives, they love the Lord, have nurtured a personal relationship with him, and attend church regularly. They have many friends, both at church and in their neighborhood. About five years ago, Denise noted that Dave was restless, and he kept asking her to repeat what she'd said. She wasn't sure if he had a hearing problem or just wasn't paying attention. He agreed to let me check his hearing, which was fine. Knowing this, Denise wasn't totally reassured and said she still sensed something was not quite right. She commented, "Perhaps work is getting to him, or maybe this is what getting older looks like." I nodded a tentative agreement but in retrospect the correct answer should have been, "Not really." As time would prove, Dave was showing early signs of dementia.

The Healthy Brain

Before we can understand dementia, we must have a basic knowledge of what a healthy brain is like as it ages. That will allow us to recognize how a normal brain differs from one that is developing dementia.

Have you ever thought much about how awesome your mind is? The very fact that we can think a thought is amazing. Our brains are packed with countless nerve cells, and the chemicals that go between those cells allow one nerve cell to affect another. This enables our brains to process and record our thoughts. But we also have immaterial souls, where our thoughts originate. Together our physical brains and our immaterial souls constitute our minds. It is like the computer I am typing on. It records and processes my thoughts, but they originate from me, not from my computer. In addition to being able to think, one of the most impressive functions of our minds is that we can remember. Isn't it astounding that, somehow, recorded in our brains are experiences we had decades ago? We can recall them in an instant, allowing the experiences of the past to impact choices we make in the present. As we begin to think about the changes in our brains that occur over time, what might impress us is not that they can fail but that they ever worked in the first place.

As our brains age, they remain capable of learning new things, recording new memories, and processing vast amounts of information. Job had it right when he said, "Wisdom is with the aged, and understanding in length of days" (Job 12:12). At times we get frustrated when our brains do not work as well as we want, and as we mature we begin to forget more things. Most commonly we struggle to recall nouns and names. We look at someone and her face is familiar, but we are not sure in what context we know her and cannot immediately come up with her name. I have found that many people who have these slips think they are getting dementia. That is usually not the case. In fact, I tell seniors that I have three types of patients: those who are normal and admit they forget, those with dementia who forget they forget, and those who lie.

One medical term used for age-related forgetfulness is "benign senescent forgetfulness" (BSF). "Benign" means it does not progress, and "senescent" means it is associated with aging. One of the important characteristics of people with BSF is that they still think clearly, not in the mental fog that so often characterizes those with dementia. I remember Janie, who, at forty, once came to the office saying that she felt she was getting dementia. When I asked her why, she cited three things: in the last week she had lost her keys, called her son by her brother's name, and forgotten something at the grocery. It just so happened that in the recent past I had done the same three things. I told her that if those were signs of dementia, she needed to get a new doctor, for I was equally demented. She laughed and continued to use me as her physician.

Normal, healthy brains can be subject to three distinct processes, the symptoms of which can look like dementia. Most common is depression. All too often elderly people get depressed in response to the losses of life. They grow more withdrawn and do not engage with life as they used to. They may appear forgetful, but the fact is, they were not paying attention to begin with. Separating depression from dementia is complicated because many people with dementia also develop depression, and there are occasions when depression is the first indication of dementia.

A second condition that may cause dementia-like symptoms is anxiety. Living in their own world of worry, anxious people's thoughts come so rapidly that they do not focus on what is actually going on around them. I remind them that a rolling stone gathers no moss. When their brains are bouncing from one worry to another, they don't take time to record things they should remember.

Depression and anxiety are both treatable conditions, yet many who suffer from them believe they have dementia.

The third condition that mimicks dementia is delirium, which is characterized by temporary confusion and agitation. This can occur with serious medical illnesses, often in the hospital, particularly in intensive care. But it may be precipitated by something as simple as a bladder infection or an adverse reaction to medications. Delirium is not dementia, though a sizable percentage of patients who experience delirium will end up with dementia.

Areas of Normal Brain Function

The human brain is a marvelous creation and is capable of many different activities. It is helpful to review these areas of neurological function, as problems can develop in any one. Think over this list, taking a moment to consider how reliant you are on your brain for each of these capacities and thank God for them:

- memory and learning
- speech and language
- intellect, including problem solving, judgment, and the abilities to recognize their cognitive problems and restrain unsocial behavior
- muscle strength and coordination
- maintaining attention
- emotions and personality
- visual/spatial ability to picture objects and mentally work with them
- executive function, which is the ability to plan and complete an activity

When we focus on memory itself, there six distinct kinds:

- immediate: grasping what we say while we are saying it
- episodic: recall of a specific incident, such as where we put our keys

- short term: recall of what occurred in the last few days or weeks
- long term: recollections that may go back to childhood
- emotional: recall of feelings long after we have forgotten why we felt them
- procedural: closely associated with muscle memory, we recall how to perform tasks such as playing an instrument or riding a bike

Even a healthy brain cannot perform all these areas of neurological function or kinds of memory with equal strength. Some of us may be better in one area than in others.

The Deteriorating Brain

Unfortunately, our brains do not always remain healthy as they succumb to the variety of diseases associated with dementia. Loss of recent memory is the most common evidence of a deteriorating brain and is likely what most people think of when they hear the word *dementia*. I remember the days of the old IBM 286 computer. It was a wonderful machine, but it did not have a fraction of the memory capacity of our present computers. It was very frustrating to go to save a document and see "Hard Disk is Full." A full computer disk is somewhat like dementia. The brain is storing many old memories, but it has no ability to store new ones. Yet, as we will see, dementia can be associated with many different problems, not simply memory loss.

First, we must understand that all forms of dementia are diseases; they are not part of normal aging. The victims cannot control what is happening to them, making it absolutely wrong to criticize or lose patience with them. When dementia gets frustrating, we must always recognize that the problem is the disease, not the person. Almost all forms of dementia can strike any person without any respect for place in society, state of physical health, or prior level of intelligence, though it is true that each of those factors can affect how the dementia impacts the victim.

Mild Cognitive Impairment

Dementia often starts with mild cognitive impairment (MCI). This is most frequently associated with a loss of short-term memory, called "amnestic MCI," and some difficulty functioning in one other area of neurologic function. Less commonly it involves not forgetfulness but dysfunction in two separate areas of brain function (called "nonamnestic MCI"), for example, difficulties in speech and personality changes. MCI will frequently lead to dementia, and though some will reverse and get better, approximately 50 percent with MCI will eventually have dementia. It is defined as dementia when people have difficulty functioning in more than two areas.

Kinds of Dementia

Alzheimer's disease. While dementia has many causes, by far the most common is Alzheimer's disease, as it causes about 70 percent of dementias. Because it is so much more common than the other causes, many people think that Alzheimer's and dementia are the same, but, as I wrote earlier, this is not the case. Once an individual has Alzheimer's, it progresses through three basic stages. In stage one the victims, though clearly compromised, can continue to live independently in their communities. In stage two they are increasingly dependent on others for help, and in stage three they are totally dependent on others, requiring help to do everything from dressing to toileting and eating. The life expectancy of a person with Alzheimer's varies widely and can range from months to twenty years; the average is in the seven-year range.

Alzheimer's typically starts with the loss of episodic and short-term memory and then spreads through the brain in a rather predictable fashion. It is like a fire that smolders and slowly spreads. The memory loss typically reverses the progression of life, so as the disease gets worse, victims increasingly lose memories in a sequential fashion. Eventually they may remember only their early childhood. At the same time patients become increasingly childlike in their behavior and dependence on others.

However, the loss of other kinds of memory may not occur at the same rate. For example, emotional and procedural memories may be more durable. I remember that in the later stages of my mother's dementia, she was unable to give my name, but her emotional memory allowed her to appreciate that I loved her, and she would expect a kiss from me. I am also intrigued that some of my patients with severe dementia are still great bridge players. They may not remember what they had for lunch, but their procedural memory allows them to win the game.

The first case of dementia was described by Dr. Alois Alzheimer in 1906, when he performed an autopsy on the brain of a woman who had developed severe memory loss in middle age, along with speech problems and behavioral changes. He found a number of deposits or plaques of what we now recognize as a substance called "amyloid," and he described how many of her brain's nerves were tangled. These microscopic changes are now recognized as characteristic of Alzheimer's disease.

But Alzheimer's is more than the physical changes that occur in the brain, for the severity of the plaques and tangles do not always correlate well with the severity of the symptoms. There are other factors that determine the impact of the disease on the victim, including how they are treated throughout their illness.

Other neurodegenerative dementias. Alzheimer's is one of a group of diseases called "neurodegenerative dementias." There are many similarities between these diseases, but in other ways they are quite distinct. They include early-onset Alzheimer's. Whereas this mimics the typical late-onset Alzheimer's in the way it affects the brain, it begins at a much younger age, between thirty and sixty, and is caused by very specific genetic changes, present from birth, that can be detected in the laboratory even before symptoms develop. It tends to progress more rapidly than many other dementias.

Another kind is *frontotemporal degeneration* (FTD), which was formerly called "frontotemporal dementia." It is characterized in its early stages more by speech and behavior changes than by memory loss. People afflicted with this disease often do things that in the past they would have known were wrong or at least inappropriate; when the disease takes hold, they fail to recognize or simply don't care that they are acting wrongly. Another tragic characteristic of frontotemporal is that the victim is unaware that he has a problem. He thinks everything is fine. This disease typically afflicts people at a younger age than Alzheimer's, and FTD has a shorter life expectancy. MRI scans show typical changes in specific parts of the brain, which allows for a more definitive diagnosis. Not all patients with FTD present the same way, as there are at least three different forms of this disease, some having more impact on language (primary progressive aphasia) and others on personality.

People with *Lewy body dementia* typically start with signs of dementia and later develop signs of Parkinson's disease. They will often experience visual hallucinations, and the disease may vacillate over time with intervals of less confusion.

Unlike Lewy body dementia, the *dementia of Parkinson's* behaves more like Alzheimer's and will be a later development in patients already diagnosed with Parkinson's.

There are other causes of dementia besides progressive neurodegeneration. Among these are vascular dementias. Representing the second-most common cause of dementia, they make up about 20 percent. Vascular dementias are caused by circulation problems in the brain, possibly one large stroke or a series of small strokes. For this reason it tends to progress in a stepwise fashion and may not show the slow, steady, predictable deterioration seen with Alzheimer's. The memory loss may be patchier and not progress from recent to long term as seen with Alzheimer's. When caused by a series of small strokes it is often associated with the heart rhythm disturbance known as "atrial fibrillation."

Dementia pugilistica is seen after recurrent brain injuries and is often associated with football players and boxers.

Encephalopathies are injuries caused by metabolic insults to the brain. Three causes are potentially correctable: deficiencies of thyroid hormone, Vitamin B1, and Vitamin B12. Encephalopathies may also be related to prolonged periods of low oxygen, as seen in chronic lung disease, obstructive sleep apnea, or severe, prolonged anemia. They can also be seen in diabetics, who frequently have low blood sugar. Other causes include years of alcohol or drug abuse.

With *infectious dementias*, we think of HIV/AIDS, Creutzfeldt-Jakob disease, or the late effects of syphilis.

Genetic disorders can also trigger dementia. Chief among these is Huntington's disease, which is passed genetically and is manifested by uncontrolled muscle movements and dementia. It is often first evidenced in early middle age.

Structural problems in the brain can also cause dementia. Subdural hematomas, where blood accumulates between the skull and the brain, can at times present as dementia, as can certain brain tumors. One other cause of dementia is *normal pressure hydrocephalus* in which there is enlargement of the fluid cavities within the brain. This typically causes dementia along with urinary incontinence and a distorted (ataxic) way of walking.

As you may surmise, determining the cause of dementia can be complicated since it is fairly common for an individual to have more than one type of dementia, and not every case fits comfortably into one diagnostic category. These are called *mixed dementias*. For example, someone with Alzheimer's may also be suffering from vascular or Lewy body dementia.

Now that you have some of what you need to know about the various causes of dementia, I will explain in the next chapter how we doctors diagnose it.

Prayer

Heavenly Father, now that I know more about healthy and diseased brains, I want to thank you for the miracle that my brain is. Don't let me waste the years I now enjoy with a clear mind but help me to serve you and be engaged in your work on this earth. As I learn more about dementia I pray that I will use this information to help others and thus bring you glory and honor. Amen.

3

What about Diagnosis?

I find that making a diagnosis of dementia, though not always straightforward, is often easier than knowing *when* to make that diagnosis. When the diagnosis is made, it provides an explanation for a number of things that may have been upsetting to the patient and family. It allows them to accept the forgetfulness and behavior changes they see as a result of the disease rather than blaming the orneriness of the victim. Early diagnosis also allows for earlier initiation of treatment. If medications could give a profound benefit, this would be a compelling argument for early diagnosis, but as we will see, such is not the case. Nevertheless, most people dread dementia, recognizing that it is a progressive disease with little room for optimism. I have seen some lose hope and give up all efforts to live successfully with dementia once the diagnosis is confirmed. It is critical for physicians to weigh the pros and cons of particular cases carefully before talking about dementia with the patient. Raising the question of dementia may or may not be helpful. The following stories may enable you to understand this dilemma.

Three Stories

Dave

While Denise came regularly to the office for her annual checkups and occasional minor illnesses, I first met Dave when he came in for the hearing check I mentioned earlier. It was several months later that Denise was in the office and said, "After you checked Dave's hearing, you said that his lack of attention and restlessness could just be normal aging. Now it is getting worse, and I am not sure it is normal. Our whole relationship has changed; we argue a lot, and he never wants to do anything fun. He worries about everything, and it drives me nuts."

I urged that they make an appointment to come talk with me about what was going on. When I saw them, I asked Dave how things were going, and he nonchalantly said he was fine. After I inquired about his state of health in a number of areas, I asked about his memory. He acknowledged that he'd been forgetting a lot of things but then said, "So does everybody else." I asked him to give me an example, and he told me about driving to the grocery store to pick up some things for Denise, but when he got a few blocks from home, he forgot where he was going, so he turned around and went home.

After I suggested that this was more than normal forgetfulness, he grunted his agreement. I did a complete medical exam and then asked my assistant to give him what I call a "mini IQ test." Taking less than five minutes to complete, this test consists of a list of thirty questions that assess various aspects of brain function. Dave's score was 22/30, clearly in the abnormal range. Faced with such a score, I may have, in some cases, immediately talked about dementia. But with Dave, I refrained from doing so because I sensed Dave was not ready for such a discussion. I felt that he might find it totally defeating and quit trying to help himself. Instead, I suggested that we have some other tests done to complete his full health evaluation. I stressed that I wanted him to stay healthy for a long time.

In addition to the routine tests I do during a physical, I included blood tests for thyroid and Vitamin B12 levels, looking for treatable causes of dementia. I also ordered an electrocardiogram and an MRI scan of his brain, again looking for treatable causes for his memory loss. At the end of the visit I told him that I agreed he had a memory problem and listed that as a diagnosis but was careful not to use the term *dementia* and certainly not the dreaded term *Alzheimer's*. I stressed we would do everything possible to help him deal better with his memory problems. I asked him to schedule a follow-up visit in two weeks. Three days later, when I had all the test results, I called to congratulate him on the tests. They looked good. I said I was still concerned about his memory, so I did want to see him for a follow-up.

That visit was difficult. Both Dave and Denise were demonstrably anxious about what they would learn. I started by asking if together we could ask for God's wisdom before we started talking, which they were glad to do. After praying, I went over the test results and then said, "Now that we know what is not causing your memory loss, we need to talk about what is." Dave spoke up, "Does that mean I have Alzheimer's?" "Dave," I responded, "We cannot say for sure, but it certainly may." Dave started to tear up, and looking at Denise he said, "Well, I guess it's all over." I took his hand and said, "Dave, we don't know what the future holds, but we do know that God is still in control. You may face major changes, but I will assure you there are still going to be happy days ahead, days when you will feel the love of your family, perhaps even more than you do now, and days when you will experience God's love and care."

Thankfully, Dave soon learned to accept his situation and cope with it by writing reminders to himself and disciplining himself to put things such as keys in a place where he could later find them. Denise was no longer upset with Dave's memory lapses and did not blame him for ignoring her. Together Dave and Denise realized they could still live enjoyable lives, which in the end made me glad that I had made the diagnosis when I did.

Sadie

Sadie's story, however, was quite different. She was brought to the office one day by her daughter, who told me they had come to talk about her forgetfulness, which was getting worse. Sadie started to cry and told me she feared she was getting Alzheimer's, as her father had had. It sounded to me as if her memory problems were fairly minor, and though she agreed with me, she repeatedly said, "I just don't want to get like Dad." After I did a brief physical exam, I suggested that she, too, have the mini IQ test. Her score was 27/30, not a great result but acceptable for someone in her seventies. I told her that we would follow her over time, but at that moment there was no evidence that she had Alzheimer's. Even as I spoke, she kept shaking her head from side to side, disagreeing with me and repeating, "I didn't get a perfect score. I knew something was wrong." Though I did my best to reassure her, she left the office unconvinced.

Afterward, she became severely depressed and experienced a total personality change. Before, she had been active, golfing several times each week and attending events at the senior center and church. Now she refused to leave the house. When her friends asked why, she told them it was because she was getting Alzheimer's. Hearing this, they eventually stopped calling and literally forgot about her. It turned out that three years later, Sadie was indeed diagnosed with Alzheimer's. As I look back, I wish I had not done the little memory test; Sadie was not helped by it.

Ernest

Another of my patients, Ernest, responded to the diagnosis with anger and denial. Always a man in control of his life, he had spent his career as a productive research scientist. He had since retired and was getting increasingly forgetful. In addition, he was becoming more domineering over his wife and often rude and abusive to his friends. Several times he had gotten lost while driving by himself and then had a series of minor fender benders. When he came with his wife to see me, I asked what I could do for him. After pointing to his wife, he replied: "Don't ask me—I'm fine. She made me come, so ask her." After she described the recent changes in his memory and behavior, she asked if I could tell him to stop driving. Ernest became noticeably upset. I was able to proceed and did a physical exam. At the end, I asked him if he would allow my assistant to give him a mini IQ test. His score was dramatically low at 15/30. I told him that the score indicated he had significant memory problems, so I was going to order several other tests to see if we could get to the root of the problem. In the meantime, I told him he should not drive. He stomped angrily out of my office, telling me I was out of my mind.

Just a week later I treated him as an emergency patient for a broken wrist sustained in yet another car accident. At that time I told him I would have to contact the department of motor vehicles to cancel his driving privileges. He became livid and rushed out of the office, swearing at me. He never saw me again and chose another physician. I later learned that he lived out the remaining two years of his life at home, being cared for by his wife. As I look back over Ernest's story I acknowledge that his life would have been happier had a diagnosis of dementia not been made, but we had no choice, for it was putting the lives of others at risk.

Each of these patients had totally different experiences, and together they illustrate the variety of ways individuals respond to the diagnosis of dementia. We now need to consider how the diagnosis is made, and then we will come back to some practical suggestions as to when diagnosis should be pursued.

How Is Dementia Diagnosed?

It is not always easy to distinguish the early stages of dementia from the forgetfulness associated with normal aging (BSF). The symptoms of dementia typically begin very slowly. Because of this, they may not be recognized as a problem until the disease is rather advanced. There are other reasons for delayed diagnosis as well. One is that because dementia is such a feared disease and can have such devastating consequences, patients and those close to them can live in denial about the disease. Not wanting to admit dementia, those with symptoms or those who see them in a loved one might initially try to attribute the symptoms to a different cause. Stress, fatigue, anxiety, depression, hormonal changes, and poor hearing are among the host of alternatives.

Another common reason for delayed diagnosis is that victims become adept at covering over their memory lapses. They tend to answer questions in general ways to avoid acknowledging that they cannot remember details. I recall that my mother always had general answers to my questions. If I asked what she had been doing that day, she would typically say, "About the same as every other day." Mother closed our conversations by saying, "Well, whatever you are going to do today, I know you will do your best." Mom had already forgotten the plans I had just shared with her. I knew that she used such tactics to conceal her forgetfulness and did not make an issue of it. Her sentiments were sincere and well intended, and I could accept that.

The diagnosis of dementia becomes even more problematic when everyone but the patient recognizes the problem. To some extent, denial represents a psychological defense, for all of us want to hold on to the life we have enjoyed as long as possible. Denying dementia is one way in which we attempt to do that. In other cases it seems that the dementia itself keeps the victim from recognizing the problem. The part of the brain that should sense something is wrong does not work. Denying dementia is rarely helpful, for it frequently makes the enjoyable life we are trying to prolong frustrating not only for the patient but also for friends and loved ones.

When we begin to suspect dementia, the Alzheimer's Association gives us ten early signs and symptoms to watch for:

- memory loss that disrupts daily life
- challenges in planning or solving problems

- difficulty completing familiar tasks at home, at work, or at leisure
- confusion with time or place
- trouble understanding visual images or spatial relationships
- new problems with words in speaking or writing
- misplacing things and losing the ability to retrace steps
- decreased or poor judgment
- withdrawal from work or social activities
- changes in mood or personality[7]

None of these changes alone is sufficient to diagnose any of the dementing illnesses, and to an extent any one of them can be caused by other factors, including other diseases, stress, depression, or fatigue; yet when one or more of them truly impacts the patient's quality of life or that of his loved ones, dementia needs to be considered.

If you are concerned about dementia, I suggest you start with your family or primary care physician, one specializing in family practice, internal medicine, or geriatrics. The doctor will want to take a detailed history of the problem from the patient and someone who knows him well. That in itself may yield the most useful information to make the diagnosis. Along with the history, the doctor will probably do a general physical that includes some type of cognitive evaluation, such as a mini IQ test, to get some measure of the extent of the problem. If a diagnosis of dementia is suspected, the doctor will order blood tests, an electrocardiogram, and possibly an MRI, CT, or PET scan to help determine the exact cause of the dementia and see if there are treatable causes.

Such tests are not necessary to diagnose dementia itself. Other laboratory and psychological tests are available and may be helpful in early diagnosis, perhaps even before symptoms develop. One form of PET scan can quantitate the amount of amyloid in the brain. This test may predict the onset of Alzheimer's years before symptoms develop, though its accuracy is not perfect. I find these tests to be of limited value. My attitude will change as more effective treatments become available. Finally, we must recognize that in the case of Alzheimer's, the diagnosis is rarely conclusive, and it is most frequently categorized as "possible" or "probable." Historically the only definitive diagnosis is made on the basis of a brain biopsy but, thankfully, this is rarely necessary.

Early-onset Alzheimer's represents a unique challenge. This condition is transmitted through the genes, which are present from birth, and these genetic abnormalities can be detected at any age by blood analysis. I feel that such testing should be offered to the children of those who carry the gene and may well already be evidencing early-onset Alzheimer's. If they are found to carry the gene, it is proof positive that they be affected. The challenge is that this disease has many levels of severity. Some who carry the gene may live a near normal life expectancy with minimal impairment. Others may be severely affected as early as age thirty. In early-onset Alzheimer's there are clearly pros and cons of doing the test, and I understand why many choose not to have it. I do not think I would want it myself.

When Should Dementia Be Diagnosed?

I have discussed some of the advantages and disadvantages of diagnosing dementia. Now it is time to be totally practical, forget the theory, and ask when *is* the right time to diagnosis dementia?

The psalmist prays, "Make me know my end" (Ps. 39:4). His point is that he wants to recognize that his life is fleeting and that he will die someday. He does not mean that he really wants to know what his last days will be like. Nor do I. I know they will end with my being in the presence of God; that's all I care to know. I do not want to know what will happen between now and then, and particularly I do not care to know if dementia is in my future. I am not even sure I want to know I have dementia until it gets to the point where I could potentially harm someone else.

In my own practice I try to determine on an individual basis when to make a diagnosis of dementia. Some patients or their families are in great distress, frustrated by living with someone with early dementia. They are upset when the same question is asked twice, let alone over and over again. They worry about the patient's safety. In these situations they can be helped by knowing the diagnosis. Others nonchalantly accept it as the normal process of getting older, and they seek to change the lifestyle of their loved one to match the decrease in mental capabilities, such as restricting driving.

Some patients, as we have seen with Dave, are helped by a definitive diagnosis, and some, like Sadie, are harmed. When I do proceed with the diagnosis, I have learned that my choice of words often determines the way patients respond. For example, talking about "a memory problem" is not nearly as threatening as using the word *dementia*, and that word in turn strikes less terror than *Alzheimer's*. Though I always want to be totally honest and forthright in communicating with my patients, this is one diagnosis about which I may compromise. I will meet with the patient and family and talk about a *memory problem*. I may then speak separately with the family and explicitly use the term *dementia* or even *Alzheimer's*.

Regarding my own health care, I admit I wrestle with when I would want to know if I am developing dementia. I plan to have regular checkups that will include blood tests for Vitamin B12 and thyroid, for if there is a deficiency here, it is much better treated before it leads to dementia than after. Since the medications available to treat dementia or delay the progression of symptoms may be most effective in early stages, I may be wise to seek early diagnosis and treatment. If, on the other hand, I would not want to try the medications and later become more forgetful, but no one is harmed by it, I hope my wife and family will be patient with me, not become overly frustrated, and let me go my merry way. However, if my condition starts to frustrate others or put them at risk, then by all means I want to be tested to determine if I have dementia. I trust that their frustration will turn toward the dementia rather than toward me and enable them to compel me to stop any activity that could endanger others. I am grateful (though somewhat intimidated) that my employer requires extensive cognitive testing for its physicians as they get older, before they are allowed to continue to practice medicine.

What Needs to Be Done after Diagnosis?

Upon diagnosis patients and their family need to sit down with the physician to have an open and forthright discussion. They need to learn about the kind of dementia they are dealing with—its cause, prognosis, and available treatment options. It is particularly crucial for the doctor to stress that there can still be a meaningful and enjoyable life in the future of someone with dementia. It is helpful to assure those afflicted that they are not crazy, that they are the same person they have always been, and that their family will love and support them. Loved ones need to be assured that the victim is still the one they have known and loved, even though he or she may be different. It must be frankly acknowledged that because there will be losses for everyone involved, it is permissible to grieve and, even at times, to experience anger and frustration.

Perhaps next most urgent is a meeting with extended family members and close friends who are willing to be involved to discuss patient care. I love to remind people that this is the time the word *family* should be a verb. Family is not something we are but something we do. If at all possible, the burden of decisions and care for the dementia patient should be shared by as many as possible even though it is usually best for the patient to have one person as primary caregiver and decision maker. I have seen some families try to move a parent with dementia from house to house every month or so, but that only promotes more confusion and disorientation in the patient and has been a disaster. But even when one person is the primary caregiver, others can do other tasks such as laundry, housework, and managing the finances.

Some of these tasks can be done even at a geographical distance from the patient. It is also wise to make arrangements to relieve the primary caregiver for several hours every week and several days each month.

If the patient has not already done so, now is the time to make sure he or she has a legally designated, durable power of attorney for medical decisions. All states allow these, though the laws that govern them vary from state to state. States also have various names for these decision makers, including "surrogate," "proxy," "health representative," and "health advocate." Clearly it is best for patients to specify who should make medical decisions when they are not capable of doing so themselves. This decision maker should be willing and available to serve, someone who knows the patient's wishes and values well and is capable of making difficult decisions. The right person will hopefully make the same decisions the patient would make if capabilities allowed. This is referred to as "substituted judgment" and is only possible if the patient has clearly communicated those wishes before becoming intellectually compromised. The appendix of this book contains a letter that I have written to my family, which you may find helpful as a starting point for such a discussion, and perhaps you will want to write your own letter.

If the decision maker does not know the patient's wishes, then a "best interest" determination can be made consistent with what is perceived to be best for the patient. Most states provide "power of attorney" forms on the Internet. Search "advance directive" online and then enter the name of your state. In addition to a power of attorney, it may also be appropriate to prepare and sign a living will and, when appropriate, a "do not resuscitate" order, which in many states is termed POLST (physician order for life-sustaining treatment). All these documents should be discussed with the physician and copies of the documents entered into the medical records.

The next step for a patient, after diagnosis is made and while there is still a degree of mental capacity, is to have a lawyer draw up documents that give supervision of the patient's finances to someone else. I remember my dear friend Liz, who, early in her dementia, was swindled by a phone scam and ended up losing thousands of dollars. That could have been prevented had Liz given one of her children financial control.

My father was a faithful supporter of a number of Christian institutions throughout his life. As his dementia increased, some "friends" who were avid supporters of a political party convinced him to give large sums to their favorite cause. We are grateful that he had appointed my sister to cosign all the checks he wrote. She was able to intercept them and significantly reduce the amount donated to the political groups, which allowed him to continue supporting the causes that had been his lifelong passion.

Along with medical and legal preparations Christians need to prepare spiritually for dementia. They should discuss the diagnosis and current needs with their pastor or other spiritual leader. All involved need to be reassured that God still loves and cares. If the diagnosis has been made public, the church ought to be praying regularly for both patient and caregivers. It may also be helpful to ask if the church could assign someone to help coordinate care in the future as different needs arise. Finally, the pastor may be able to put victims and their families in touch with others in the congregation facing similar challenges for mutual encouragement, prayer, and sharing helpful hints.

One real dilemma is to decide whom to inform of the diagnosis. There is an unavoidable social stigma associated with this disease, leading some to shy away from those with dementia or even cut them off. On the other hand, those not informed about someone's dementia may be insensitive and rude to the victim. I suggest that at the very least, those who are in close contact with the patient should be informed, including those in the service industry such as a hairstylist or servers at an oft-visited restaurant. This prepares people to interact with the dementia sufferer in an appropriate way. Others will not need to be informed of someone's dementia diagnosis unless the behavior of the patient startles or frustrates them. Often, a quiet "Please excuse us—we have a memory problem" from the caregiver will suffice, and the word will get around. The Alzheimer's Association recommends having an information card printed that briefly explains the condition and can be discreetly given at such awkward moments.

Prayer

Heavenly Father, I feel like I am starting to travel through a foreign country where I do not know the language and do not know how to act. It is clear that I need wisdom that can come only from you. Without your help I am lost, so lead me by your Spirit. And in whatever way dementia is going to impact my life, I pray that I respond in a way that will honor you. I pray this for my good and for your glory. Amen.

4

Can Dementia Be
Prevented or Treated?

Now that we have explored issues involved in diagnosis, it is time to consider what help is available. We will start with some medical options and then consider more personal ways to help.

As Dave and Denise learned to cope with Dave's dementia, I encouraged them to attend two support groups, one for patients with early dementia, as Dave had, and one for caregivers like Denise. Unfortunately, these groups met 50 miles from their home. They attended a session but then decided that the benefit of participating did not outweigh the difficulty of the long drive through heavy city traffic. Instead, they began to take regular walks together and continued to eat a healthy diet, and Denise found some games they could enjoy together. I also started Dave on two medications, one for the dementia and one for depression. After several weeks Denise noted that Dave was not crying as much and was not quite so dependent on her; however, she did not feel that it helped his memory to any significant degree. Thankfully, their insurance paid for the expensive medications, and Dave tolerated them well.

Ways to Impact All Dementias

The bad news, as you will see, is that currently there is no known way to improve the microscopic changes in the brain that cause the most common dementias. The good news is that there are means to help reduce the impact of dementia and so improve quality of life for both patient and caregiver. Ways to help all dementias include the following.

> *Exercise.* Thirty minutes of physical exercise at least five days a week can improve the circulation to the brain and is one way to reduce falls, which people with dementia are at increased risk of.

> *Diet.* Eating a diet heavy in olive oil, nuts, and veggies, while low in red meats and saturated fats (a Mediterranean diet), will benefit those with dementia, just as it would all of us. It may be particularly helpful in preventing vascular dementias. Many advocate particular vitamins and supplements to help dementia, but though most do no harm, there are no studies that confirm long-term benefit, and they may potentially interact with other medications. Vitamin E has been shown in some studies to have some limited benefit.

> *Medications for coexisting conditions.* Depression is often associated with dementia, and using an antidepressant such as sertraline (Zoloft) or citalopram (Celexa) can be of significant help. Closely associated with depression and yet quite different is the apathy of dementia, which does not respond to antidepressants but may do better with a stimulant such as methylphenidate (Ritalin).

> *Vision and hearing.* Correcting vision, including the removal of cataracts, and improving hearing with the use of hearing aids keep us more connected to the world around, which is critically important for those with dementia. Needless to say, it is very hard to remember what we cannot see or hear. Im-

proved hearing may aid with memory, and it can stimulate the brain in other ways as well.

Social involvement. Those who are socially involved and focused, not on themselves but on others, do better than those who are isolated.

Spiritual lives. Those who continue to practice their religion, attend church, and maintain their spirituality have been shown to cope better with their mental limitations.[8] A regular prayer life can become part of one's procedural memory and persist well into dementia.

Using the brain. It is common sense to keep using and strengthening the parts of the brain that still function well. Doing activities such as crafts, knitting, and crossword puzzles or other word games can help. Reading and watching TV may be of value only if you take time to write or discuss your reactions. Otherwise they are simply passive activities that do not require much thought.

Maintaining a regular schedule. Getting up in the morning, going to bed at the same time each night, and eating meals at the same time help some.

Respecting the dignity of those with dementia. Setting forth the dignity of every human being is the basic premise of this book and one of the most effective ways to improve life for those with dementia.

Conversely, there are a number of lifestyle practices that can make dementia worse, as follows.

Stress and sleep deprivation. Simplifying life to reduce stress and getting proper rest can delay the progression of dementia.

Smoking. This not only increases the risk of stroke and the vascular dementias but may lead to lower oxygen levels in the blood that further damage the brain.

Alcohol. Drinking alcohol is toxic to brain cells, and since it goes more readily to the aging brain, it is particularly harmful to those with dementia.

Overtreating blood pressure or diabetes. This may lower the blood flow to the brain or the blood sugar that the brain needs.

Chronically low oxygen. Low oxygen levels, whether from lung disease, sleep apnea, or anemia, have been shown to accelerate dementia in some people.

Anesthesia. Certain anesthetics may lead to a sudden drop in blood pressure, contributing to brain damage.

Medications. Some medicines are commonly associated with worsening cognition. The worst offenders are tranquilizers and sleeping pills. I will acknowledge, however, that there are times when the behavior of those with dementia becomes so disruptive that sedatives are necessary to safeguard them from harming themselves or others. If a sleep aid is needed, I often recommend melatonin or the antidepressants trazadone and mirtazapine.

Most drugs prescribed for urinary incontinence have also been associated with worsening cognition, as have antihistamines, which often produce drowsiness. Statins are a cholesterol-lowering class of drugs that may occasionally make dementia worse, but the benefits—including minimizing the chance for vascular dementias—far outweigh the risks. Some tricyclic antidepressants may also make dementia worse, as can alpha-blocking blood pressure medications.

Travel or hospital stays. Events that disrupt the daily routine, including any kind of overnight travel, are disorienting and often upsetting to those with dementia.

Mistreatment. Treating anyone, including those with dementia, in demeaning or insulting ways is a surefire way to aggravate cognitive problems.

Degenerative Dementias

As I mentioned earlier, degenerative dementias—including Alzheimer's, Lewy body, that of Parkinson's disease, and frontotemporal degeneration—are the most common. Regarding Alzheimer's, we must understand that what appears to be the basic underlying cause, plaques and tangles in the brain, has been developing for as long as twenty years before a patient is symptomatic. Those of us who attempt to treat Alzheimer's are frustrated that medical science offers no solution to curb the development of these microscopic changes. However, there are some promising drugs currently being evaluated that may do that.

After the plaques and tangles are well established, it is believed that they are the culprits that begin to kill nerve cells and lead to a deficiency of the chemicals called "neurotransmitters," whose job it is to carry signals from one cell to another. A deficiency of these chemicals may further promote nerve cell death. Only after this process has gone on for some time (years) do the symptoms of dementia become evident. Currently prescribed dementia medications work by increasing the amount of neurotransmitters in the brain. Because they do not get to the root of the problem, I often liken them to calling the bomb squad after the explosion. That being said, there are certain cases when they do seem to help, and even if they do not, they may slow the progression of the disease. For this reason they are often worth trying, and if tolerated by the patient, it is reasonable to continue using them.

Currently there are two classes of medications approved by the Federal Drug Administration (FDA) available for treatment of dementia. The first class is termed "cholinesterase inhibitors." These include:

- Donepezil (Aricept), the only drug approved for all stages of dementia.
- Galantamine (Razadyne), approved for mild to moderate dementia.

- Rivastigmine (Exelon), also approved for mild to moderate dementia. This drug comes as a pill or a patch, which is convenient for those who have trouble swallowing pills.

All these cholinesterase inhibitors are fairly expensive and can cause stomach upset, frequent stools, and slow heart rate. In some cases, these drugs do not lessen memory problems but do minimize some of the unwanted behaviors associated with dementia, which can certainly justify their use.

The second class of medications, called "memantine" (Namenda), works in much the same way but affects a different neurotransmitter and so can be complementary to the cholinesterase inhibitors. Side effects of Namenda include headache, confusion, constipation, and dizziness. It is approved for patients with moderate to severe dementia and sometimes provides additional benefit when taken with one of the cholinesterase inhibitors.

In addition to dementia drugs, antidepressant medications may help the patient feel better and reduce some of the emotional outbursts and sleep disturbance that can occur in the course of the disease.

Apart from Alzheimer's, the other forms of degenerative dementias do not respond as well or even at all to these medications. There is some evidence that rivastigmine (Exelon) may be beneficial for those with Lewy body dementia, particularly those who experience visual hallucinations. Frontotemporal dementia does not respond to any of these medications but may do better with the antidepressant citalopram (Celexa).

Vascular Dementias

More options exist for those with vascular dementias. Stroke prevention treatments reduce the risk of vascular dementia, and these include lifestyle changes and medications to manage blood pressure, cholesterol, diabetes, obesity, sleep apnea, and stress. Recognizing and treating atrial fibrillation is a way to prevent vascular dementia. Atrial fibrillation occurs when the upper chambers of the heart (atria) stop beating as they should, allowing clots to form in them. At times those clots can break up and travel to the brain, where they cause a large stroke or a series of small, often undetected strokes. As small strokes accumulate, they can lead to dementia. The incidence of those clots can be reduced more than 50 percent by taking a blood thinner like Coumadin (warfarin) or one of the newer products available. Simply taking an aspirin each day will somewhat reduce the risk of these blood clots. The effectiveness of Alzheimer's drugs on vascular dementias is unclear. When it comes to vascular dementias, there is no question that an ounce of prevention is worth a pound of cure.

Other Dementias

Treatment options for some of the other causes of memory loss that look like dementia are more hopeful. Neurologic problems caused by low levels of thyroid hormone or Vitamins B1 and B12 can be dramatically slowed and often significantly improved by appropriate replacement therapy. Subdural hematomas can be surgically evacuated. Normal pressure hydrocephalus can in certain cases be helped by surgically inserting a shunt to drain the excess fluid. Many of the infectious causes can be treated. Unfortunately there is no medical treatment for the causes of some dementias, such as Huntington's.

Spiritual Resources

I would be remiss to leave this discussion of dementia treatment without mentioning prayer, a privilege we as Christians have when facing the challenge of any illness: "Is anyone among you sick? Let him call for the elders of the church, and let them pray over him, anointing him with oil in the name of the Lord. And the prayer of faith will save the one who is sick, and the Lord will raise him up" (James 5:14–15). God is interested in our physical, mental, emotional, and spiritual healing. The individual suffering from dementia needs our prayers for all of these. Whereas the passage in James singles out church elders to pray, it does not limit prayer to just the elders; all believers should pray for the healing of others. God may not always answer our prayers by changing circumstances; sometimes he responds by changing our attitude toward those circumstances and graciously allowing us to get through them.

Prayer

Heavenly Father, as I confront dementia, I am fully aware that there is little I can do to control the disease itself. I am thankful that my life is in your hands and that I can trust you. I pray that I will have wisdom to take advantage of the treatments you have provided, but I know they will not do anything unless you are in them. I am grateful that the ability to cure is in your hands, and if it be your will, I pray for that. If not, I pray for the ability to cope and that this dementia would accomplish your sovereign purpose, for I know that you are loving and strong. I pray this for my good and for your honor. Amen.

5

How Does It Feel to Have Dementia?

Our God is compassionate, and we, too, must be compassionate. Compassion is not only showing love and kindness, but it is also understanding how others feel and then allowing ourselves to feel that same way. It is taking the time and effort to get into their lives to see the world as they see it. If they are frustrated, for example, we must allow ourselves to feel that frustration. This is crucial when relating to those with dementia. Ask yourself what it would be like to waken every morning with a full bladder but be unsure of where you are or where the bathroom is. And imagine how you might feel if someone who seems only vaguely familiar begins to undress you. And how would you feel if you wanted to say something but all your words came out as unintelligible gibberish? You would feel horrible, of course. No wonder those with dementia get frustrated, start to cry, or burst out in anger. As a way of fostering compassion, I want to give you a glimpse into what having dementia feels like.

Dave and Denise learned to live with frustration. One of the early changes Denise noted in Dave was irritability, especially when they were doing more than one thing at a time. If they were having a conversation while the television was blaring in the background, Dave got very upset because he could not focus on what Denise was saying. Dave also got angry whenever he misplaced his car keys. He tried to remember to place his keys on the hook by the door, but he occasionally forgot and put them in his pocket. Later he would think someone had taken them from the hook. Once Dave even accused Denise of hiding the keys to play a trick on him. Denise tried to understand and cope with a growing list of idiosyncrasies. Dave began to cling to her, wanting to be with her most of the time, as he felt increasingly uncomfortable facing new situations and unfamiliar people. Valuing her own space and desiring to have some time by herself, Denise did not take Dave's desire to be with her as a compliment.

Dave recognized that he was changing, and he knew something was wrong. At times he could talk through his frustrations; at other times he couldn't. He would just sit and cry. It was not easy, but to her credit Denise tried patiently to sit down with Dave, hold his hand, and ask him how he felt. Talking with her occasionally made him feel better, and he often forgot what had been bothering him. As Denise became more familiar with dementia, she became more compassionate, for she began to see the world through Dave's eyes.

Emotions of Early to Mid-Dementia (Stages 1 and 2)

To foster our understanding and compassion for the person with dementia, it is helpful to first consider the different experiences and emotions of those in the early and mid-stages of the disease. This will put us in a better position to respond positively to them.

One characteristic of dementia is how constricting it can be. Before the onset of dementia, victims live in a big world. They are concerned with some of the events taking place around the globe; they enjoy getting out and traveling to different places. They are conscious of history and intrigued at how events of the past impact the present. They also know that what happens in the present will affect the future, and such awareness helps determine the choices they make. With the onset of dementia, their personal world begins to shrink and they become less concerned about events in the larger world. They are quite happy to remain in their hometown, which shrinks to their neighborhood and then to their home and eventually to one room. Similarly, they don't remember or care about the past and no longer care about the future. Eventually they think only about themselves. We may think, "How sad! Consider how much they are missing." But it doesn't seem to bother them as much as it does us. They still have the capacity to enjoy the present, and without other things to compete with that, the here and now becomes all the more important to them.

It is also critical to understand the emotions often associated with dementia, which I have had plenty of opportunity to observe. Clearly not every person with dementia exhibits similar responses, but I've listed below some of the emotions to watch for. I write these as if you were the person with dementia to help you feel what it is like.

Alienated. Your friends respond to you differently. They don't talk to you the way they used to and don't ask you to do things with them anymore. You assume they no longer like you.

Apathetic. You have made so many mistakes and embarrassed yourself so often that you can easily get to the point where you no longer care. You would rather sit and do nothing than try and fail.

Bored. Set aside from a busy, productive life, you are not able to accomplish anything. Life is boring.

Depressed. There is little that makes you happy. You cannot remember the last time you really felt well.

Dominated. You were used to making a lot of decisions and were able to control most areas of your life, but now you cannot. While you resent others taking control, deep inside you know you need help and appreciate them taking over.

Embarrassed. You were always pretty sharp, but now you make a lot of mistakes. You know your problems are obvious to others, yet you can do nothing about it, so you would rather withdraw from people to avoid the embarrassment. When asked to do something, you refuse because you are afraid of failing.

Fearful. You recognize that something terrible is happening to you, and it frightens you. Fear has become part of your daily experience; there are so many things going on around you that you do not understand. You hear loud noises and, not recognizing what causes them, you worry something will hurt you.

Frustrated. You forget so many things and are unable to learn new information. You have thoughts and want to express them but cannot organize sentences or find the right words. You feel like crying.

Hopeless. In the early stages of dementia, when you are still aware of the diagnosis and its prognosis, you recognize that it will only get worse, and it is hard to find any basis for hope.

Ignored. Life is going on all around you, but you are just sitting there. People speak to you, but they say things so fast that you cannot understand them, and they don't take time to listen to you. They don't seem to care.

Inattentive. You can no longer concentrate. When you read, you cannot retain the material, nor can you follow a story on TV.

Irritable. So much happens that you do not understand, and it irritates you. You get mad at someone you know is trying to help, and that irritates you all the more. Somehow you recognize that this is not "you," but you cannot seem to control it.

Lonely. You want to withdraw from others, yet you miss being with people. You still desire the presence of others; you want to feel respected and loved. You desire to be touched, hugged, and kissed, but you frighten some people, and they do not appreciate that you have these needs.

Meaningless. Your life used to be filled with meaningful activities that contributed to the world around you, but now that is all gone.

Suspicious or paranoid. You cannot find something you are sure you put in a certain place, and you think someone may have stolen it. You hear people talking but cannot recognize what they are saying and suspect they may be talking about you.

Other Changes in Early Dementia

One question I am commonly asked is how much of an individual's personality prior to the onset of dementia is carried over into their dementia. We discussed earlier that some healthy people are more independent, while others are more dependent; some are more joyful, and others more sullen; some are trusting, while others are suspicious; some are extroverts, while others tend to want to be on their own. Whatever the traits of our pre-dementia personality, there are likely remnants that will persist as dementia progresses. It may also be true that the lack of inhibition associated with dementia allows some previously suppressed aspects of our personality to come out in unexpected ways. If we were calm and loving, we may become boisterous and even hateful. If we were typically trusting of others, we may become suspicious and paranoid; and if generally happy, we may become old grouches. Fortunately, sometimes the opposite occurs and formerly frustrating characteristics are shed or become easier to live with.

One variable that profoundly affects the way people experience dementia is their level of insight as to the nature and extent of their impairments. Some people are keenly aware of their deficiencies and need a lot of sympathy, love, and encouragement. They may be able to honestly discuss their situation and express their frustrations, which allows them to benefit from a support group and be open to suggestions for ways to improve their situation.

Others, lacking insight, will be oblivious to their problem and go on their merry way, thinking that everyone else in the world has a problem, but certainly not them. Such lack of insight is particularly associated with frontotemporal degeneration. In such cases, it's not a matter of simple denial but a part of the disease itself; the part of the brain designed to recognize memories, judgment, and behavior simply does not work. Those who lack insight need safeguards for their safety and that of others they may be putting at risk. Additionally, they are unlikely to benefit from a support group, nor will they be open to discussing their situation. Those retaining insight are much harder on themselves; those without insight make it much harder on others.

Many grieve the losses incurred with dementia. The loss of productivity along with many relationships, independence, and even some memories can lead to grief. Some with dementia can also go through periods in which they freshly grieve an old grief. Lourdes had lost her mother twenty years earlier and had grieved appropriately. When she developed dementia, she would ask for her mother and when told that her mother was dead, she would go into hysterical grief all over again.

There may be stages in the grief of dementia similar to those that Elisabeth Kübler-Ross observed in terminally ill patients.[9] These include denial, bargaining (trying to do something to affect the outcome), anger, depression, and then, at times, acceptance. The stages do not necessarily progress from one to the next; each can be experienced at different times. Dorothy and I observed these stages as her mother progressed through dementia. Initially she would deny that she had a problem and was quite determined to continue to live independently as she had till that point. Later, when we felt the time had come for her to leave her home in St. Louis and move to an assisted-living facility near us in the Chicago area, she understandably became quite angry. This was followed by a period of depression in which she did not want to do things or initiate conversations. In her later months, however, she became more accepting of the fact that she had dementia and the changes that accompany it.

As Christians we should also be interested in how dementia affects people spiritually, even from the earliest stages. In this regard each individual has a unique story. There may, however, be common themes. Some will begin to question God's love and power. They may ask, "Why me?" and question whether God has any purpose in what they are experiencing. They typically lose the vibrancy of their daily walk with God. Concentrating at church, in their Bible reading, or in group discussions may be more difficult. They may become spiritually discouraged. Others, fortunately, will recognize their dependence on God and will learn to trust him on a deeper level.

The Experience of Moderate Dementia

As dementia progresses, sufferers may be less conscious of their deficiencies. Even so, many of the emotions experienced in early dementia are still present. At the moderate stage there might also be delusions during which things and events are misinterpreted. A sound in another room might be attributed to the presence of a burglar.

I remember when my mother, in a delusional state, thought that I was my father, a fairly common delusion. Others may believe they are in their childhood home. Delusions differ from hallucinations, which might also occur at this stage, in which the individual may see or hear things that are not there. In one sense, delusions and hallucinations may not be much different from dreams or nightmares, the difference being that they occur when the patient is awake.

The spiritual experience of those with moderate dementia is

similar to that of those in the earlier stages, only more severe. Pastor Robert Davis offers us some insight from the chronicle of his journey through dementia, which he wrote with the help of his wife. Prior to dementia, he'd had a close and fulfilling experience with the Lord for his entire adult life. But as his dementia progressed, he became terrified by waking at night to a "blackness" in his mind. It was not only an inability to feel God's presence; he felt nothing. He wrote: "Now I discovered the cruelest blow of all. This personal and tender relationship that I had with the Lord was no longer there. This time of love and worship was removed. There were no longer any feelings of peace and joy."[10] But that was not the end of the story. He continues: "By sheer stubborn faith, I knew that God was there and that Christ was my Savior. However, the feelings that I had enjoyed all my life were gone." Later he recounts how the Lord did answer his prayer. One night he seemed to hear the Lord's voice say, "Take my peace. Stop your struggling. It is all right. This is all in keeping with my will for your life. I now release you from the heavy yoke of pastoring that I placed upon you. Relax and stop struggling in your desperate search for answers. I will hold you. Lie back in your Shepherd's arms and take my peace."[11]

Conversely, some dementia victims experience spiritual benefits as the dementia worsens. Long-held guilt over past sins and a corresponding struggle to accept God's forgiveness in Christ are forgotten. Those beset by constant anxiety and worry are freed from the tension as they become less aware of the world outside. In some cases dementia can contribute to a believer's victory over sin and in that sense serve to purify their conscience. Sinful thoughts that earlier in their lives intervened in their communion with God become less prominent. God may also use dementia to free them from memories that do not honor God, including pride taken in personal accomplishments. If pride has kept them from humbly accepting God's grace, the humility of dementia enables them to find new peace in God's unconditional love.

Severe Dementia

In all honesty, we do not know much about what it's like to experience severe dementia because victims are unable to share how they feel. People at this stage lie in bed, rarely showing any response. Though they may put together words, those words rarely make sense and offer no clue about what is going on in their minds. We are left only with questions: Are they thinking thoughts that make sense to them even though they cannot express them? Do they understand what we say to them? Can they feel loved by those caring for them? Are they even aware of others around them? Do they have any consciousness of God? Is the Holy Spirit still a source of comfort? We have no answers to these questions, and if we did, those answers would likely vary from person to person and from time to time.

Though we can only speculate, it is reasonable to think that those with severe dementia are not terribly conscious of their plight. They are likely not bothered by their incontinence or other things that would previously have embarrassed them. I suspect that it is much more distressing to observe a person who has severe dementia than to be the one who has it.

Some with severe dementia have an emotional peace and will occasionally respond with a smile or nice words such as "I love you" or "thank you." I remember being touched during home visits to Felecia. Her daughter would stroke her arm and say, "I love you, Mom." Felecia would say, "I love you too, Sweetie." This happened many times a day, but each time was beautiful. Ruth was quite the opposite. Though prior to dementia she was just as kind and loving as Felecia, once in decline she would push her daughter away rudely, saying, "Don't touch me." I wish I knew what had been going on in Ruth's mind.

For the most part, though, persons even in the most severe stages of dementia seem to do better when others pay attention to them, demonstrating that they are still social beings. They still value pleasant experiences such as eating tasty food, so this may be the time to forget a healthy diet and allow them to enjoy the foods they crave. They also appreciate good aromas and may be offended by the odors associated with their incontinence. They like viewing beautiful scenes and enjoy the closeness of someone reaching out to touch them.

Patients with severe dementia will often sit and do nothing, which can be disturbing to their loved ones. This is not an indication that they are thinking troublesome thoughts; most likely they are not thinking at all.

I know this is not a pretty picture of the experience of dementia, but I trust that it is helpful for you to know just a bit of what it must be like. The goal of this book is to help us understand how God can be honored through the experience of dementia, and one of those ways is for us to truly feel what it must be like to suffer from this disease.

Prayer

Father, I get a sense of how very difficult it can be to experience dementia. If that is what you have for me in my future, I pray that I will have your grace to come through in some way that will honor you. I never want to disgrace your holy name. And if your call to me is to care for someone with dementia, I pray that daily I will have some sense of what his or her life is like so that I may be truly compassionate. I pray this for my good and for your honor. Amen.

6

The Experience of Caregiving

The patient is not the only victim of this dreadful disease; caregivers are just as much, if not more, affected by it. As we must understand what it is like to be the victim, so we must understand what it is like to care for a person with dementia. As we understand more of the caregiving experience, we will develop some compassion for caregivers. We will see that providing loving care to a victim of dementia is one of the key ways in which this complicated disease can honor God.

Challenges for Caregivers

Just as there is a wide range of the ways victims experience dementia, there is a wide range for the ways it impacts the lives of the caregivers. Earlier we talked about the good, the bad, and the ugly for those with dementia; so it is for their caregivers. You may find this chapter difficult, for I am not painting an altogether happy picture of caregiving. But don't be discouraged! In the next chapter we will talk about some ways to make it better and to see caregiving the way God sees it.

Denise is a good example of what it's like to be a caregiver. As Dave progressed through his dementia, I was impressed that he actually looked fairly well. Dave appeared rested and no longer cried as he had earlier; however, Denise looked increasingly fatigued and stressed. On the occasions when Dave did get upset, Denise would reach out to touch him. It seemed rather sweet and romantic, and he would visibly relax at her touch, but Denise would utter an almost imperceptible sigh, with a look of frustration on her face. I began to notice that she was rather sharp in her responses to Dave.

During that same period, I saw her more frequently at the office for various minor illnesses, viral infections, and stomach problems. She would tell me how Dave clung to her most of the time, catnapped a lot during the day, and wandered around the house at night. She scarcely had a moment to herself, was suffering from sleep deprivation, and was falling into a severe depression. She told me several times that she had asked her children to come stay with Dave so she could get away for a while, but they always had other things to do. Sympathetic to her situation, her pastor put a message on the church's electronic bulletin board, asking for others to stay with Dave for short periods, but none offered the help she desperately needed.

Denise's experience is all too common. Consider the statistics on caregiving. There are approximately eight million Americans with dementia (five million with Alzheimer's). Of these roughly 70 percent live at home, and 75 percent are cared for by their families or friends. Most often, the caregiver is either the spouse or the daughter or daughter-in-law. Serving a loved one with dementia is never what anyone would choose, yet caregivers often serve at great personal sacrifice.

Challenges from the Patient

The challenges faced by caregivers vary from day to day and from one case to another. Though there is no stereotypical case of dementia, we can identify some of the behaviors that typically challenge caregivers.

Anger. Patients with dementia can exhibit anger, particularly with the ones they depend upon the most. I have often wondered why. Perhaps it is the contempt of familiarity. Perhaps the caregiver's presence reminds the patients of how dependent they are, and they resent that. Perhaps they are tired of being told what to do, for, like any of us, they do not like being bossed around. Perhaps there is difficulty adjusting to role reversals between parent and child or within a marriage. Perhaps it is all these and other reasons as well. From a personal standpoint, my mother-in-law was always pleasant to me, but she vented her anger on my wife, Dorothy, who loved her dearly and cared for her so well. Dorothy described her mother's behavior with others as her "social behavior."

Vacillation. Day-to-day change in patients with dementia can be frustrating for caregivers. Patients may have good days and behave almost normally, but on other days they are totally confused, uncooperative, and downright cantankerous. Provoked caregivers wonder, "Why couldn't she do today what she did so well yesterday?" Conversely, there are times when the patient seems to have some level of control. I recall two situations in which two loving daughters cared for their mothers, both of whom had moderate dementia and were increasingly uncooperative and difficult to manage. Both daughters had brothers who lived far away and rarely had contact with their mothers. In each case the sisters pled with the brothers to come and visit to better understand what was going on. Thankfully, the brothers finally came, but in both cases, the mothers put on their best behavior during the visit, leading the brothers to believe that their sisters were blowing the problem out of proportion. Someone with dementia can do well for a brief visit from a loved one but cannot keep it up long-term. It takes a lot of effort to force a deteriorating mind to keep up its social behavior. Additionally, the sons, during their short visit, did not have to give the sort of care the sisters provided on a daily basis that their mothers found so demeaning.

Lack of appreciation. Persons with dementia rarely acknowledge the sacrifices their loved ones make for them. It is truly a thankless job. It is not just those with dementia who rarely say thank you, but also other family members who are not carrying their share of the load. They will fail to express appreciation if they assume the caregiver is simply doing her duty.

Apathy. Those with dementia often lack the motivation to get up and get going, which can prove frustrating for caregivers.

Loss of inhibition. We all think bad thoughts occasionally and have impulses to do what we would otherwise recognize as inappropriate, crazy, or even evil. Fortunately, a healthy brain recognizes those thoughts as wrong and dismisses them. I recall with horror my friend Hugo, a quiet, unassuming academic, who, for no good reason, drove through four stop signs. When pulled over by the police, he argued that what he'd done was perfectly safe since there were no cars coming. Were it not for a call to his wife and her explanation of his decreased mental capacity, his lack of inhibition would have resulted in arrest. It did, however, end his days of driving. The patient's lack of inhibition can be embarrassing to the caregiver, which in turn can limit social encounters for the patient, thereby contributing to social isolation for the caregiver.

Slowness. Everything a caregiver does with a dementia patient takes more time than expected. Whether it is dressing, eating, or going to the bathroom, the caregiver's patience is required.

Accusations. Dementia patients can easily assume that problems stemming from their dementia are the fault of someone else. Unable to find a wallet or purse, the caregiver is accused of stealing.

Communication. It can be painfully difficult to grasp what those with dementia are trying to say and to make sure they understand what you are saying to them.

Shadowing. As we noted earlier, those with dementia can feel insecure and fearful if left alone. This dire need for security makes them want to know their loved one is close by, which rarely allows the caregiver a moment of solitude.

Meltdowns. When feeling totally confused, patients can lose all control. The resulting meltdown is similar to the temper tantrum of a two-year-old. Those with dementia may become verbally or physically abusive and a threat not only to their own safety but to those around them as well. Meltdowns can be triggered by any number of things. Among the most common are overstimulation, being startled, or tiredness. Though there might be warning signs of an approaching outburst, allowing for the possibility to avert it, other times they go full-blown, requiring the caretaker to drop everything else to calmly and lovingly soothe the victim.

Sundowning. People with dementia typically become more confused and agitated late in the day. Just when the caregiver gets ready to unwind and relax after a full day, the patient requires even more attention and effort.

Sleep disturbance. Having dementia often inhibits one's ability to get adequate restful sleep, which causes physical and emotional problems that the caregiver must deal with. In turn, the caregiver sleeps no better. This is usually most difficult in the later stages of the disease, when the patient reverses days and nights. It is further complicated when the victim wanders or is severely agitated at night. This was the case with Eleanor. Although in a later stage of dementia, her husband continued to care for her in their apartment. One very cold, predawn morning she was found walking outside in her nightgown. Under God's watchful care, a neighbor spotted her, called her husband, and got her to the hospital. Miraculously Eleanor was unharmed, and she returned to her home. Unfortunately, that was the end of restful sleep for her husband until Eleanor's condition eventually required her to be placed in a nursing home.

Making messes. People with dementia make messes; they spill their food and can be incontinent. They fall and get hurt, or knock things over and break things. Such messes make more work for caregivers.

Desire for meaning. Persons with dementia have the same need for meaning and fulfillment as others do. Providing for and planning activities to accomplish this goal adds one more task to the caregiver's list.

Overall, caregivers find that there is neither the time nor the energy to do everything required. One of the most helpful books on dementia care is *The 36-Hour Day* (see the Suggested Reading section for more information). The title of that book says it all. The work of a caregiver can quickly amount to more than a full-time job.

Additional Challenges

As if the challenges of personal care of the patient were not enough, there are many other hurdles to overcome. Included are the frustrations involved in dealing with the medical system. Making appointments, getting the patient to them, reviewing insurance claims, paying bills, and picking up drug refills are just a few, all of which require time and energy.

Then there are the frustrations of dealing with community-sponsored support agencies. Though intended to be of help (and they often are), they do not come in response to a simple phone call. No, there are forms to fill out—both to apply for the service and to verify financial need. Once the services start, they can be a great help, but there is often a good deal of hassle getting them going.

Not only are caregivers distressed by the burden of caring for those with dementia, but their distress is worsened by a lack of people with whom to share that burden. Other family members fail to help, as do formerly close friends. Most tragically it is often the church that fails to provide the badly needed support.

The Toll on the Caregiver

One by one, the challenges of caregiving begin to erode the caregiver's health and sense of well-being. This is seen on a number of fronts.

Physical

As dementia progresses, the physical toll on caregivers increases. Blood pressure begins to rise, and gastrointestinal problems, including hyperacidity and bowel problems, may occur. They may have insufficient time to eat or prepare a healthy diet, and they are overstressed and sleep-deprived. All this may lead to a lowered immune response, making them more susceptible to anything from colds to serious infections such as pneumonia. As patients become weaker and less mobile, the physical strain on caregivers increases and can cause chronic back pain or strains in their shoulders and other joints.

Recall James, the "ugly" case I told you about in the introduction. He was the domineering father who, while adored by his wife and daughters, was so difficult to care for when his dementia became worse. What I left out of the sad story was that the day after he was moved to a dementia-care facility, his wife was admitted to the cardiac care unit at the hospital with an uncontrolled heart rhythm. I am sure her condition was brought on by the stress of dealing with James.

One statistic I find amazing is that 30 percent of caregivers die before the patient for whom they are responsible.[12] This number of deaths cannot be directly attributed to the stress of caregiving, but it must be a contributing cause. Knowing of this physical toll, caregivers have the added burden of needing to make contingency plans for the care of their loved ones in the event that they are no longer able to provide it.

Mental

The mind of a caregiver can never rest. There are the ever-present problems of communication and finding creative responses to the needs or strange behavior of the dementia patient. On top of these moment-by-moment concerns, there is the need to think ahead about when and how to grocery shop, never knowing when patient care might prohibit a necessary outing. Can they risk taking their charge with them, or must they find someone to fill in at home while they go out alone? The answer may well vary from day to day according to how the patient is doing, which makes planning ahead difficult.

Finally there are longer-term perplexities to consider: "Will I eventually need to make arrangements for a nursing home or hire someone to help provide care at home?" That in itself is a complex choice, for though added help may provide needed relief from the burden of caring, it is hard to find the right person, and even then, someone new will need to be instructed and supervised. Other really tough questions include, "What about end-of-life decisions? Should I sign a do not resuscitate order? Is hospice appropriate?" There is no end of questions to wrestle with, which can leave the caretaker exhausted.

Social

Being a caregiver can be lonely and isolating. There is little time to get out and enjoy other activities and relationships. The pleasure of entertaining visitors in the home can be spoiled by the embarrassment caused by the victim's odd behavior. Besides, the patient may have a meltdown when overstimulated by the presence of company. These indignities may cause caregivers to stop asking people to visit, further diminishing their needed interaction with others. Imprisoned in their own home with only the patient, who can give increasingly less emotional support, cabin fever quickly sets in.

Financial

Dementia can cause havoc to the household budget, which is yet another new challenge for the caregiver. Extra expenses come in droves. It may be necessary to remodel the house to allow for a wheelchair or make a bedroom on the first floor; ramps may be needed to get into the house. Pads and special clothing may be necessary to deal with incontinence. Hiring part-time help in the home is expensive, but nursing-home care is expensive as well. All this financial outlay might come right during the loss of income of both the caregiver and the patient.

Emotional

Taking on the role of primary caregiver of someone with dementia is the most common cause of midlife depression. Almost all caregivers will have periods of sadness and discouragement and a lack of emotional resilience that add to their mental and physical exhaustion. Part of the depression is a feeling of hopelessness, caused in part by the awareness of the inexorable progression of the disease. True, after having a bad day, the one in charge of the victim can hope the next day will be better. But the caretaker is aware that such good days are numbered. Every time one detects further mental deterioration in the patient, it is a grim reminder of the future course of the disease. No wonder the situation is depressing.

Grief is also common for caregivers. Besides lamenting the loss of the meaningful relationship they once had with the patient, they grieve the loss of the happy activities and freedom they used to enjoy. When a spouse or parent slowly becomes a stranger, a major part of the caretaker's life is taken away.

As noted earlier, there will also be times of anger. Caregivers can feel anger at the patient for the frustrations they cause, anger at others for not being there to help, anger at the medical team for not providing expected care, anger at themselves for feeling angry, and even anger at God for permitting this horrible disease to come into their lives. It is essential for caregivers to be able to vent their anger in a healthy way lest it get vented on the patient. The abuse of people with dementia is all too common and under-reported.

Another emotion caretakers may have is fear. They may fear no longer being able to provide the needed care or not knowing what to do should an emergency arise. At times there is fear that the individual with dementia will have a meltdown and become violent and physically abusive. Then there is the honest worry, particularly for children who are taking care of their parents, that they will develop dementia themselves. I remember Marge telling me about that fear. Then she chuckled and said, "I guess I'd better do a good job taking care of Mom so my daughters will follow my example."

On the other hand, in spite of all of the negative emotions, there are positives, and we will develop these further in a later chapter.

Spiritual

Perhaps the highest toll for caregivers who follow Jesus is felt in their personal relationship with God. Some Christians have grown up thinking that God intends each of our lives to be easy and happy, and when that is the case, they will not likely do well facing the challenges of dementia. In addition, on a practical, day-to-day level, in the midst of their busyness caregivers may not have time or energy to read their Bible, go to church, spend time with other Christians, or pray more than a quick cry for wisdom and help. As a result, God might seem absent. They may long for him to step in and help them through their difficulties, but if they don't see it happening, they may feel he does not hear or care. They feel their plight deeply and passionately cry out to God, as did the psalmist:

> Awake! Why are you sleeping, O Lord?
>> Rouse yourself! Do not reject us forever!
> Why do you hide your face?
>> Why do you forget our affliction and oppression?
> For our soul is bowed down to the dust;
>> our belly clings to the ground.
> Rise up; come to our help!
>> Redeem us for the sake of your steadfast love!
>> (Ps. 44:23–26)

I mentioned at the beginning of this chapter that I would not be presenting a pretty picture. It is true—being a caregiver has many challenges. But not only are there ways to help make it less onerous; there are definite benefits to caregiving. In the next chapter we will consider some of these.

Prayer

Heavenly Father, I know that you are all good and all powerful. If you have entrusted me with the responsibility of caring for a victim of dementia, I pray that you will allow me to find refuge in you. I long to have your wisdom and your strength and pray that you will graciously provide so that I may learn to trust you more. As I see other selfless caregivers sacrificing so much of their lives, I pray for them and ask you to show me how I can be of practical help. I pray this for the good of your people and for your honor. Amen.

7

Help for Caregivers

Being a caregiver may have its burdens, as we've seen, but now I would like to focus on the positive aspects of serving those with dementia, including the fact that it honors God. We must remember that God has entrusted caregivers with the opportunity to serve his special creations, those made in his image, who suffer from dementia. As we engage in loving service and relationships, not only do we honor God, but we find more meaning in life, whether we are the caregiver or the victim of dementia.

Denise was a great example of a loving caregiver. Midway in the course of Dave's illness, when life at home was becoming more difficult, Denise sent me an email update. She spoke of her conviction that God had called her to love and serve Dave through his illness. "I know it won't be easy, but I will do what I know God wants me to do," she wrote. She reminded me that years earlier at their wedding, both she and Dave had vowed to care for each other "till death do us part." Denise wrote, "With God's help, that is exactly what I intend to do." She closed the email by referring to the day when both Dave and she would stand together in God's presence: "He will be healed, and we will stand together as whole persons rejoicing in God, and I will look back on the sacrifices I made down here and know that I had been given a great privilege to serve the two I love most: Dave and Jesus."

Called to Serve

Caregiving is a distinct call from God. It is not something we randomly fall into. Unfortunately, it may seem like this responsibility is foisted upon us, but that is not true. We often think of God's calling as something that comes to us through a great, supernatural experience, but often the call comes to us by the circumstances he puts in our path. If I am walking down the street and the person in front of me collapses in a cardiac arrest, my calling from God, at that moment, is to rush up and initiate resuscitation, call 911, and do whatever else I can. Believing that God made us, knows everything about us, loves us, and is in control of the details of our lives, it is only logical to trust that he knows that the experience of caregiving, with its great stress and limited joys, is just what we need to mold our character and make us like Jesus. If the opportunity for caregiving is presented, and you seem to be the logical person to serve, it is often reasonable to conclude it is God's calling for you. Once we see caregiving as a calling, it is easier to accept it as our priority and not feel guilty about ignoring other pursuits.

Unfortunately many Christians are not able to trust God so fully. In fact, I suspect that few are able to face this daunting challenge. They may never have learned that part of God's plan for their lives is to mold their character to be more like the Lord Jesus by leading them through difficult experiences.

Those who recognize caregiving as the call of a kind and loving God will hopefully respond to it, not with a grimacing fatalism but with a joyful expectation of what God is going to accomplish in their lives. James writes, "Count it all joy, my brothers, when you meet trials of various kinds, for you know that the testing of your faith produces steadfastness. And let steadfastness have its full effect, that you may be perfect and complete, lacking in nothing" (James 1:2–4).

Caregiving may be a trial, but it is carefully orchestrated by a loving God to transform the life of the caregiver. Furthermore, the caregiver will recognize that the sacrifice of Jesus on the cross was, in part, to be an example of sacrificial giving to others. That is the point Peter makes when writing, "For to this you have been called, because Christ also suffered for you, leaving you an example, so that you might follow in his steps" (1 Pet. 2:21). Jesus's charge to his disciples was, "If anyone would come after me, let him deny himself and take up his cross and follow me" (Matt. 16:24). Rather than an invitation to fun and games, we are called to sacrificial service.

It is also helpful to recognize whom we are called to serve. First and foremost we serve God. Earlier we referenced Matthew 25:40, where Jesus said that whatever we do for someone in need, we are doing for him. And Paul tells us to do the will of God from our hearts, "rendering service with a good will as to the Lord and not to man" (Eph. 6:7). But our service is not only to God, for we are actually serving one made in God's image. John Kilner writes, "The reason that people warrant love is not that people are so lovable in themselves but that love is the appropriate way to treat those in God's image."[13] It may be hard to believe that the person sitting there speaking nonsense, unable to eat or dress, and incontinent, is in fact made in the image of God, but that is the way God sees him, and so should we. In serving those particularly in the later stages of dementia, we are not only fulfilling our Lord's instructions to serve the needy, but we are giving without the expectation of receiving anything in return (Luke 6:35–36).

If you are approaching caregiving with a lot of resentment, you need to pray and ask others to pray that the Lord will change your heart and confirm to you a sense of his calling. Giving care to a person with dementia can be a catastrophe for all concerned if it is motivated by guilt or obligation rather than love and the joy that comes from doing what your Lord and Savior has called you to do. Knowing that God himself has called you to a task should bring confidence and perhaps even pleasure as you do it.

Called to Love

It is not enough simply to meet the needs of those with dementia. To honor God, we need to do it in ways that consistently reflect his love. True love is not onerous. When any task, no matter how unpleasant it may be, is done in love, it is in some way transformed. I have known many loving caregivers over the years. What has amazed me is not just that they are loving when I am with them, but that they consistently demonstrate God's love day in and day out through all the ups and downs of dementia. I must tell you, however, that it is not the default. So we should explore several characteristics of caregivers who give this type of love.

One thing I am not is a Hebrew scholar, but one Hebrew word I have come to appreciate is *chesed*. Used several hundred times in the Old Testament, it is translated as "steadfast love." Other translations may use the term *lovingkindness* since there is no exact English equivalent. It is most frequently used to refer to God's love for his people and reflects his kindness and mercy. It also emphasizes God's loyalty and commitment to their well-being. We will never be capable of loving even the most lovable on that level. The amazing thing is that God pours *chesed* love on those who are in no way lovable. This *chesed* love should be the model that a caregiver shows a victim of dementia. It is characterized by kindness, faithfulness, and mercy.

I have seen *chesed* love in many couples as they faithfully serve each other. When I have the chance to do so, I frequently ask husbands or wives caring for a spouse with dementia if this is what they were thinking of when they stood in front of the church decades earlier and promised "to have and to hold from this day forward, for better, for worse, for richer, for poorer, in sickness and in health." None has ever acknowledged that dementia was in their thoughts at that time. I then congratulate them on doing what they promised and tell them that God is pleased with their faithfulness.

A wonderful book called *A Promise Kept* by Robertson Mc-Quilkin tells the author's story of resigning as the president of Columbia International University to give himself fully to what he described as the privilege of caring for his wife, Muriel, who suffered from dementia.[14] This was truly *chesed*. I am equally impressed with the sacrifice that children make to care for declining parents. They may have to quit work and take time away from their own children and spouses, not to mention their favorite leisure activities, but they are truly honoring their parents.

Now, I do not mean to imply that every moment of every day will flow out of a loving heart, but the general tone should be motivated by love. Remember that true biblical love is often expressed most fully in responsible behavior and self-sacrifice. The greatest love the world has ever known was when Jesus submitted himself to the will of the Father and went to the cross.

Look to God to Enable Loving Care

Each stage of dementia has unique challenges in providing loving care. From the repeated questions and forgetfulness seen in the early stages to the lack of communication and need for total care in the later stages, there is a daily strain. But the good news is that God himself is a caregiver's caregiver. He will give daily strength, wisdom, love, and patience. Take a few moments to reflect on these Scriptures:

> It is my prayer that your love may abound more and more, with knowledge and all discernment, so that you may approve what is excellent, and so be pure and blameless for the day of Christ, filled with the fruit of righteousness that comes through Jesus Christ, to the glory and praise of God. (Phil. 1:9–11)

> The fruit of the Spirit is love, joy, peace, patience, kindness, goodness, faithfulness . . . (Gal. 5:22)

> May the Lord make you increase and abound in love for one another and for all, as we do for you. (1 Thess. 3:12)

> God gave us a spirit not of fear but of power and love and self-control. (2 Tim. 1:7)

> Beloved, let us love one another, for love is from God, and whoever loves has been born of God and knows God. Anyone who does not love does not know God, because God is love. In this the love of God was made manifest among us, that God sent his only Son into the world, so that we might live through him. In this is love, not that we have loved God but that he loved us and sent his Son to be the propitiation for our sins. Beloved, if God so loved us, we also ought to love one another. No one has ever seen God; if we love one another, God abides in us and his love is perfected in us. . . . We love because he first loved us. (1 John 4:7–12, 19)

God will give us that love and the strength to do what he calls us to do when we do not have it within ourselves. Many of us have never truly learned to depend on the Lord and draw our strength from him. J. I. Packer writes, "The weaker we feel, the harder we lean. And the harder we lean, the stronger we grow spiritually, even while our bodies waste away."[15] It is as he provides that we are able to do anything truly good. Paul writes, "God is able to make all grace abound to you, so that having all sufficiency in all things at all times, you may abound in every good work" (2 Cor. 9:8). Peter puts much the same thought this way: ". . . whoever serves, as one who serves by the strength that God supplies—in order that in everything God may be glorified through Jesus Christ. To him belong glory and dominion forever and ever. Amen" (1 Pet. 4:11). Yes! The greatest resource a caregiver will ever find to provide loving care is God's own love and the indwelling presence of God's Spirit. These should never be overlooked.

Plan in Advance

One of the good things about dementia is that it usually progresses slowly. Once it is suspected, whether formally diagnosed or not, there is often time to prepare for it. During this time, I suggest doing several things.

Learn as much about dementia as possible. Both caregivers and patients should learn as much as possible about the disease. Some may be reading this book just for that purpose. In addition, consider getting some of the other books listed in the Suggested Reading section. Go to the Alzheimer's Association website (http://alz.org), which is filled with useful information. See if there is an Alzheimer's Association support group nearby. In some cases there may be separate support groups for patients and caregivers. Support groups for patients will be most helpful in early or mild cases, when the victims have some insight into their problem.

Pray. Start praying that God will fill you with love, wisdom, and strength for the job ahead. Recruit some close friends to faithfully pray with and for you. Ask God to remove any resentment and give you a spirit of joyful service, even a heart of gratitude for the opportunity to serve.

Spend time in the Bible. Start reading through your Bible and jot down ideas you find that may impact your role as a caregiver. Begin with the Gospels to discover in the character and work of Jesus what you desire to emulate. Ask God to use his Word to cleanse and transform your attitudes while he teaches you his values.

Assure That Your Own Needs Will Be Met

I mentioned in the introduction that it has always been my prayer to be able to serve others out of a sense of fullness rather than emptiness or looking for affirmation and praise. Frankly, living in a fallen world, it is simply not possible to always achieve that fullness and have our motivation perfectly pure and attitudes positive. Some things will exhaust us; at such times we should do our best to accept and endure them, anticipating that times of refreshment will follow. It is then that we need to practice unselfish *chesed* love—a love that is faithful, steadfast, and loyal. It is also at those times that we should begin to investigate what help is available.

There are proactive steps you can take to preserve your ability to honor God with loving care. One of these is to carefully think through the increasing strain that caregiving will bring and develop strategies for how you will maintain your capacity to serve without coming to the end of your emotional, physical, and mental strength. You must anticipate how much free time you truly need, how to assure you obtain it, and how to use it well. Remember your need for exercise as well as mental and spiritual refreshment, including Christian fellowship. Start planning early how you will be able to meet those needs as the requirements of caregiving increase.

If you fail to meet your basic needs, you will very quickly burn out, and the quality of your care will deteriorate. Your frustration will rapidly transfer to the person you are caring for. If you, in your exhaustion, become irritable, your patient will too. If you are refreshed, calm, and loving, your patient will more likely be the same way. Recognize right from the beginning that providing care for someone with dementia is not a one-person job. God is honored when we humbly acknowledge that we need help and seek it.

Learn What Hands-On Help Is Available

What type of help should be considered? There are a number of options.

In-home nursing services and home-health aides. Almost every community has home-health agencies that provide nurse visits to monitor health needs and home-health aides to help with such regular tasks as bathing, feeding, or staying with the patient while the caregiver goes out. It is ideal to introduce those with dementia to the outside caregiver early in the course of the disease to allow them to develop a relationship of trust, which will be invaluable as the disease progresses. Initially a limited commitment of, say, a half day a week will be adequate, with the idea that the level of service will increase as the needs arise. Some states provide these services with no or reduced fees for those who cannot afford them. The local chapter of the Alzheimer's Association may be able to direct you to appropriate individuals or local agencies.

One difficult decision is whether to hire an independent, secondary caregiver or secure the services of an agency. Independent helpers may be willing to provide companionship in the home twenty-four hours a day often six days a week, making your home their home. That type of arrangement is often less expensive and can be a win-win for both the person with dementia and the primary caregiver, and it allows for a close relationship of trust to develop. On the other hand, independent helpers need a fair amount of supervision, and the primary caregiver will have no backup if he or she becomes ill. By working through an agency the primary caregiver can avoid those disadvantages because the agency is responsible for supervision and backup. The disadvantage is that an agency is pricey.

Adult day-care programs. Many communities have facilities that provide daytime care anywhere from one to five days a week. Frequently housed in nursing homes or hospitals, they provide activities, socialization, meals, and basic care. The patients often enjoy time with the friends they make there, and these facilities provide a needed break for the caregiver and also enable a caregiver to work, if need be. In certain cases the facilities provide transportation to and from a patient's home. And some states and communities even provide funding for these programs. Attending an adult day-care program several days a week and having professional in-home care the other days can provide a wonderful mix of engaging activities. Making good use of such resources can lengthen the time that the dementia patient can live at home.

Assisted living. Assisted-living facilities can be wonderful options for the care of those with dementia. They typically provide a private bedroom and bath as well as large common areas. Meals are served in dining rooms. Activities are provided both on- and offsite, while 24/7 medical help is available. Many facilities have special areas designated for patients with dementia, and some are totally dedicated to dementia care. The nursing and support staff are well trained to handle dementia patients and to enrich their lives. Medicare does not pay for assisted living, and it is rarely covered by state-run public aid programs. When specific requirements are met, long-term health insurance or the Veteran's Administration will pay some of the costs.

Nursing homes. Nursing homes are often viewed as a last resort. Indeed, in many cases they should be. Yet they have a role. Nursing homes run a wide spectrum in the quality of care they give dementia patients, some being excellent and others considerably substandard. All will provide meals and activity programs along with basic nursing care and services such as dressing and feeding those who require such help. Unfortunately the cost of quality nursing-home care is so high that most families can manage to pay only for a short time. After that, the state public aid program ("Title 19") often steps in, though what they pay is rarely adequate to cover the bona fide expenses of excellent care. Top-rated nursing homes often do not accept patients on public aid, and those that do are often understaffed. I have worked in some of these facilities, and whereas sometimes I grieve the care given, I have the utmost respect for the staff who do their best with limited resources. Nursing homes also accept patients with dementia for short-term "respite" stays to give the caregiver a break. This may be covered by Medicare if the patient is on hospice.

The local church. I am convinced that a local church is one of the most underutilized resources available to Christian caregivers. It is so critical that we will explore it in more depth in a later chapter.

When Is It Time to Get Help?

God calls us to be good caregivers, but he also knows our limitations. As the psalmist says, "As a father shows compassion to his children, so the LORD shows compassion to those who fear him. For he knows our frame; he remembers that we are dust" (Ps. 103:13–14). There are limits to what a caregiver can do even with God's help, and God does not expect us to exceed them. There may be a temptation to push beyond those limits. Some try to be a superhero while others develop a martyr complex. Feeling sorry for themselves, they stubbornly try to slug it out even though they have lost all the joy that giving care once provided and feel totally drained physically, emotionally, and spiritually. Insisting on going it alone when depleted is not honoring to God or in the best interest of the patient or caregiver.

But there may also be good reasons for caregivers to resist asking for help, such as a lack of other qualified caregivers who know as much about the patient or would be so loving and careful. True though that may be, any caretaker must recognize that the quality of their own care will start to diminish. Caregivers must limit the expectations they put on themselves and ask for help when it is needed. Older caregivers may be limited by their energy levels, physical strength, or diseases, including their own cognitive abilities. Younger caregivers may be limited by competing responsibilities such as the care of their own families or a job and may need help sooner.

Obtaining help should be a gradual process that starts from the early days of dementia. A good place to begin is talking with experienced caregivers and learning from them. Later, as the needs progress, help in the home might be required, starting with a half day a week and increasing as the needs of either the patient or the caregiver become greater. Such help may come from a trained professional or a family member or a loving friend. When starting as a caregiver, it is best to take the attitude that help will be necessary. It is not a question of *if* but *when.*

There may come a time when home care is not enough, and the difficult decision to pursue residential care is in the best interest of both victim and caregiver. One indication that the time has come is when caregivers have lost joy and feel spiritually dead, emotionally drained, and mentally or physically exhausted. Deep in their soul, they know they are not providing the type of care their loved one needs, and they become conscious that their motivation is no longer love but obligation and perhaps a little bit of stubbornness. In this case, it is time to pursue residential care if possible, and it may be the only recourse left for following Paul's exhortation to "not grow weary in doing good" (2 Thess. 3:13). Moving to a nursing home or similar facility becomes not a sign of weakness but of the strength to do what is right.

The other person to consider in this decision, of course, is the victim of dementia. He may be at the point where he has no appreciation for the sacrifices being made to keep him at home. It's important for caregivers to know that after the patient adjusts to new surroundings, he might be equally content to live in a facility. In fact, he may actually be happier having others around. The move to a nursing home may be much harder on the caregiver than on the patient. If, on the other hand, he continues to derive obvious pleasure from being at home, other sources of help should be pursued and nursing-home placement deferred.

The final group of stakeholders in the decision to pursue residential or nursing-home care is children or teenagers in the home whose needs might require a higher priority than the wishes of the person with dementia.

I am particularly sensitive to the emotional state of caregivers who promised in the past that they would never place their loved one in a nursing home. I typically ask caregivers if they are able now, before the condition worsens, to have a rational discussion with their patient about reconsidering the earlier promise to avoid nursing-home care. Most of those I ask acknowledge that their loved one would likely release them from the promise, willing to sacrifice their own pleasure for the good of their caregiver and other family members. The story is told of a gentleman coming to his last days with dementia. In one of his rare lucid moments he asked his wife, "Has this torn the family apart?" When she said, "No, it has brought us closer together," he responded, "Oh good."[16]

Apart from the caregiver's exhaustion, there are other situations that may precipitate admission to a long-term care facility. Most frequently it is an acute illness involving hospitalization, or a fall with a fracture that dramatically increases the patient's care needs. Because the need for nursing-home care may be urgent, it is advisable for the caregiver to take time before the need arises to explore what options are available and choose a facility. It is best to choose one that offers a continuum of care so that future deterioration will not require a move to a different facility. Many people find that nonprofit facilities, perhaps run by a church or other religious organization, are best. Additionally, I have observed that nursing homes in a rural setting offer better care than those in an urban context. We were amazed at the loving care Dorothy's sister received over a number of years in a facility in a strongly Mennonite community.

Caregivers' lives will be dramatically changed once the patient has moved to a chronic-care facility. But even then, they must still be intimately involved in their loved one's care, visiting often and continuing to advocate for them. Caregivers won't typically have to complain to the staff, but their very presence and loving attention to the patient assures more attentive care for their loved one. This is one more way to honor God through dementia.

Once the transition to a residential care facility has been made, whether nursing home or assisted living, caregivers may feel guilty and burdened by a sense of failure even though they have done their best. These feelings are rarely appropriate and can lead to depression that persists long after the move has been made and even after the death of the patient.

What Are the Rewards for Caregiving?

Tough though it may be, providing loving care for a victim of dementia can still be rewarding. We do well to consider first the rewards offered in this life and then, as believers who have the hope of eternal life, we look to those that will come in eternity.

Rewards in This Life

Knowledge that you are doing what is right. Caregivers know that providing good care is the right thing to do, even when part of them rebels against it. When it is all said and done and the patient's life is over, I have often heard caregivers say something like, "Well, it was tough, but I am glad I did it."

Following in the footsteps of Jesus. The Lord Jesus is our greatest example of unselfish service. The prophet Isaiah presents him as the "suffering servant." Jesus spoke of his own call to serve even at great price to himself, "for even the Son of Man came not to be served but to serve, and to give his life as a ransom for many" (Mark 10:45). Caregivers should derive great pleasure from knowing they are doing what Jesus would have done.

Jesus taught us that we should serve others without looking for a reward ourselves. We may find that particularly true when we serve those with dementia. One of the more challenging sayings of Jesus is, "Love your enemies, and do good, and lend, expecting nothing in return, and your reward will be great, and you will be sons of the Most High, for he is kind to the ungrateful and the evil. Be merciful, even as your Father is merciful" (Luke 6:35–36). I do not believe that the patient with dementia is our enemy (though the disease itself is), yet if this is the way we are to treat an enemy, how much more should we serve such a person, even without the anticipation of reward in this life?

God's transforming the caregiver's character. God does not waste his or our time. He has purpose in everything he brings into our lives. One of his purposes in dementia is the refinement of the character of the caregivers, using the disease to transform them to be more like Jesus and so bringing honor to our Lord. This is so important that we will come back to it later.

Growth in trust. As we grow in our Christian experience through overcoming the challenges of life, we learn to rely more fully on the presence of the Holy Spirit within us. We become more conscious of his love and wisdom consistently working through us, and this allows us to trust him more.

Affirmation from the patient. Even in late-stage dementia victims will show the occasional sign of recognition and appreciation for the care they are receiving. My mother, even in great confusion, would occasionally convey her appreciation with a smile and softly say, "Thank you" or "I love you." These expressions of gratitude did not occur often, but each time they did, they were immensely meaningful to me.

Eternal Rewards

We have seen that when we do things for others in need, Jesus views it as actually doing it for him. That is a privilege and may be reward enough. Providing loving care is doing God's work, and that lasts for eternity. Paul writes, "Therefore, my beloved brothers, be steadfast, immovable, always abounding in the work of the Lord, knowing that in the Lord your labor is not in vain" (1 Cor. 15:58). This is written in the context of our ultimate resurrection from the dead, so "not in vain" means that it will yield eternal consequences.

The results of loving care will be seen in eternity, and there will be rewards in heaven that will make those received in this life pale in comparison. The primary motivation to provide loving care should not be what we get out of it; God, in his righteousness and justice, will see to it that we will not go without our due reward.

We basically have three options for how we spend our time: we may choose to invest time well, doing things with eternal value; we may spend most or part of our lives in sin; or, third, we may spend time doing things that, though not bad in themselves, are frankly a waste of time. There will come a day when we will stand before God to have our works judged. Thankfully, we will not be judged for our sinful deeds, for when we trusted Christ, they were forgiven. What will be judged is the amount of time we invested in doing good for eternity in comparison to the time we wasted. Paul compares our good deeds to gold, silver, and precious stones, whereas time wasted is wood, hay, and stubble that will go up in smoke:

> Now if anyone builds on the foundation with gold, silver, precious stones, wood, hay, straw—each one's work will become manifest, for the Day will disclose it, because it will be revealed by fire, and the fire will test what sort of work each one has done. If the work that anyone has built on the foundation survives, he will receive a reward. If anyone's work is burned up, he will suffer loss, though he himself will be saved, but only as through fire. (1 Cor. 3:12–15)

Without question, the loving care provided for patients suffering from dementia will be part of the gold, silver, and precious stones that will be rewarded in eternity. Caregivers will be among those who hear the wonderful phrase: "Well done, good and faithful servant. You have been faithful . . . enter into the joy of your master" (Matt. 25:23). Yes! God is honored when we unselfishly provide loving care to those who cannot repay us. One of my favorite hymns from a bygone era says it so beautifully:

> O Love that wilt not let me go,
> I rest my weary soul in thee;
> I give thee back the life I owe,
> That in thine ocean depths its flow
> May richer, fuller be.
>
> O light that followest all my way,
> I yield my flickering torch to thee;
> My heart restores its borrowed ray,

That in thy sunshine's blaze its day
May brighter, fairer be.

O Joy that seekest me through pain,
I cannot close my heart to thee;
I trace the rainbow through the rain,
And feel the promise is not vain,
That morn shall tearless be.

O Cross that liftest up my head,
I dare not ask to fly from thee;
I lay in dust life's glory dead,
And from the ground there blossoms red
Life that shall endless be.[17]

God's call to care for a person with dementia is a huge challenge but in many ways a wonderful opportunity. It requires a deep humility to recognize that we cannot do it ourselves. But thanks be to God, help is available, and we need to seek it when needed.

Prayer

Heavenly Father, I know that at times you call us to things that are very difficult. I am grateful that your purpose is not just to give me a happy and secure life. Your purpose is to honor yourself by doing a work of transformation in my soul. I submit my life to you as a living sacrifice and pray that you will use it to honor your name. Give me the strength to do what is right and to share your love with others in whatever way you desire. I pray this for my good and for your honor. Amen.

8

How Can We Honor God through Dementia?

We come now to the heart of this book: honoring God in and through the tragedy of dementia. We have considered biblical foundations, reviewed what we need to know about dementia, including its diagnosis and treatment, and gotten a bit of a feel for what it must be like to experience dementia both as a patient and as a caregiver. The key question to ask is, if God's purpose in all things is that he be honored and glorified, how does a tragedy like dementia fit into his larger scheme? The next question we must ask is, what steps can we take to be part of God's plan and honor him through dementia? We will discover there are a number of ways. God is honored when we:

- Embrace biblical values
- Respect the dignity of those with dementia
- Meet the needs of dementia patients
- Provide loving care
- Involve the church
- Grow through the experience
- Pray, trust, and place our hope in Christ
- Come to the end of life well

Value What God Values

Let's go back to Dave and Denise. Dave's dementia was slowly progressing. The times when Dave would respond positively to Denise were getting fewer. He still wanted to be with her, but rarely did he want to hold her, and sometimes he was unable to say her name. He seemed to view her as a friendly stranger. He did not keep track of the day and rarely wanted to leave the house. Denise felt she had lost her best friend. Not only did she miss Dave as her husband and lover, but she felt she was losing Dave as a companion. If she tried to read to him, he could not follow and sometimes rather rudely told her to stop. After discovering he still enjoyed listening to music, she played his favorite albums for him, especially recordings of old hymns. She found other ways to give him pleasure, such as serving him a bowl of ice cream. When he started to cry, she learned to stop what she was doing, sit beside him, and hold his hand. She commented to me that although he did not seem to be the person he once was, he was still a person who deserved her love. Denise confided that as much as she loved Dave, she was ready for the Lord to take him home. She was looking forward to the day when he would be healed and together they could enjoy eternity with Jesus. Denise was learning to value what God values.

If we are going to honor God in and even through dementia, we first need to know God in an intimate way. We need to think the way he thinks, respond to life's situations the way he responds, love the things he loves, and value the things he values. When we know God in this way, we are able to respond to dementia the way God himself would respond.

We have already seen the need to appreciate that dementia was not a part of God's originally good creation but came as a consequence of sin. We need to understand that God is in control and has purpose in everything he allows and does, including dementia. Thankfully, we see in the cross of Christ and in our salvation how God takes bad things and turns them around for good. Though it may be difficult to accept, he can do the same with dementia. Finally, we appreciate that our eternal home is not this world with all its challenges and sin; our destiny is to be in God's presence. This includes both the ones who suffer from dementia and all those involved in their care. Our trials will be over and we will find peace, rest, and ever increasing fulfillment in God's presence.

What truly gives our lives value? Stephen Post has insightfully written:

> We live in a culture that is the child of rationalism and capitalism, so clarity of mind and economic productivity determine the value of human life. The dictum "I think, therefore I am" is not easily replaced with "I will, feel, and relate while disconnected by forgetfulness from my former self, but I am." . . . Human beings are much more than sharp minds, powerful rememberers, and economic successes.[18]

When we buy into the myth that our intellects and abilities define our worth, we do two things wrong. First, we take on a false sense of our personal value, and, second, we diminish the value of those who lack those same capacities. We demean one made in God's image, and in that sense we desecrate God himself. It's almost like throwing dirt on a picture of those we love. We must always keep in mind that dementia is a disease. When people are suffering from pneumonia, we do not expect them to be able to accomplish what they did in health, and we do not question their worth. So it should be when the affliction is dementia.

There are several corollary questions we should address.

Are those with dementia still whole persons? Earlier I said that a person was the intrinsic union of body and soul. Here I want to emphasize that it is not necessary for both body and soul to be perfectly well to render someone a whole person. Too often I have heard healthy people refer to those with dementia as "half persons," or "bodies still alive after the mind has died." It is true that dementia may significantly alter a personality, but it does not alter the fact that they are persons. They may behave differently, but they are still whole people. All those born to human parents are human persons made in God's image. We must treat them as persons, not as objects. To use the terminology of philosopher Martin Buber, we must relate to them in terms of "I-thou," not "I-it." Dementia may compromise the awareness of the self, but it does not diminish the self.

Does God love and value persons with dementia? He certainly does, as we noted earlier. God said, "Behold, all souls are mine" (Ezek. 18:4). This is an all-inclusive statement that makes no distinction between those with dementia and any others, for all are souls. One of the best-known verses in the Bible is John 3:16, where we read, "God so loved the world," which means he loves everyone. God sees all of us as broken and in need of his love. How we are broken doesn't matter.

How much does God value our intellect? The answer is—not as much as we do. Perhaps the apostle Paul puts it best:

> For consider your calling, brothers: not many of you were wise according to worldly standards, not many were powerful, not many were of noble birth. But God chose what is foolish in the world to shame the wise; God chose what is weak in the world to shame the strong; God chose what is low and despised in the world, even things that are not, to bring to nothing things that are, so that no human being might boast in the presence of God. And because of him you are in Christ Jesus, who became to us wisdom from God, righteousness and sanctification and redemption, so that, as it is written, "Let the one who boasts, boast in the Lord." (1 Cor. 1:26–31)

The prophet Jeremiah would agree:

> Thus says the LORD: "Let not the wise man boast in his wisdom, let not the mighty man boast in his might, let not the rich man boast in his riches, but let him who boasts boast in this, that he understands and knows me, that I am the LORD who

practices steadfast love, justice, and righteousness in the earth. For in these things I delight, declares the LORD." (Jer. 9:23–24)

While we may want to think highly of our intellects, God doesn't. We do well to remember the teaching of Jesus: "So the last will be first, and the first last" (Matt. 20:16). Our conclusion must be: God values those with dementia and we should too.

God Values Emotions, Feelings, and Relationships

God values our emotions, for he, too, has emotions. We read of him rejoicing (Isa. 62:5), loving (Ps. 103:17; Isa. 54:8), grieving (Ps. 78:40; Eph. 4:30), being wrathful (Ex. 32:10), and having pity (Ps. 103:13). He is concerned not only about how we think but also about how we feel. He created us to experience joy, love, and pleasure, but he also gave us the ability to be angry, depressed, and discouraged. These emotions are just as much a part of our being whole persons as our cognitive abilities.

In addition to having feelings, God responds to pleasant sensations; he is depicted in the Bible as one who hears, smells, and appreciates beauty. One of the beautiful images of heaven is of Jesus sitting down with his bride at a banquet. Banquets are a feast for all our senses—seeing, hearing, tasting, smelling, and feeling. He created us to enjoy them all. Our emotions and our ability to feel things are just as much a part of our being full persons as our intellect. Emotional and sensual pleasures are not lost with the progression of dementia.

Finally, God is relational. Throughout eternity past, God has existed as one God in three persons. When he created mankind he said, "Let us make man in our image, after our likeness" (Gen. 1:26). (Note the plurals.) Prior to the creation of Eve, God said, "It is not good that the man should be alone" (Gen. 2:18). Although that was spoken in the context of marriage, it need not be restricted to the marriage relationship. God created us as social beings needing relationships with others.

Since God included emotions, sensual pleasures, and social relationships as distinctive features of our humanity, we must never discount the value of those who, although lacking cognitive abilities, can still experience emotions, enjoy feelings, and benefit from being around others.

God Values the Present Moment

One way in which we as human beings are not like God is our relationship to time. We are confined to the present moment. We experience one instant, and then it is gone, never to be recaptured except in our memories. We may wonder what the future holds for us, and though we may trivially say, "God only knows," that is in fact true. God, while able to enter time and travel through it with us (as did the incarnate Jesus), also lives in all of time in the present tense. If you put all of history on a timeline, God would be present over the entire length at the same time. If you have trouble understanding how that can be, you are in good company—I do too. But consider these passages:

God said to Moses, "I AM who I AM." (Ex. 3:14)

Before the mountains were brought forth,
   or ever you had formed the earth and the world,
from everlasting to everlasting you are God. (Ps. 90:2)

Jesus said to them, "Truly, truly, I say to you, before Abraham was, I am." (John 8:58)

For thus says the One who is high and lifted up,
   who inhabits eternity, whose name is Holy . . .
      (Isa. 57:15)

I love the way Isaiah says that God "inhabits eternity." When God is called "I AM," the use of the present tense indicates that from eternity past to eternity present, he is ever present.

There are times when I love to simply enjoy the present moment. I can pull away from the past, stop thinking about the future, and allow myself to be consumed by the present. Dorothy and I love to take walks at sunset, drinking in the beauty of the moment. At those times, nothing else seems to matter; we enjoy the present. Perhaps that is somewhat like God, for he, too, values the present. Dementia's victims also do this, especially as their disease progresses. They no longer worry about the future and become less and less conscious of the past. By finding peace and joy in the present, they are not concerned about their loss of memory and other capacities.

Scripture and Memory

Since much of dementia is about memory, we need to give some thought to how the Bible views our ability to remember. In the book of Deuteronomy alone, the word remember occurs fourteen times, and in the ESV overall, the words remember, *remembrance*, *memory*, or *forget not* occur a total of 226 times. Just for example consider Psalm 103:2: "Bless the LORD, O my soul, and forget not all his benefits." Or Deuteronomy 32:7: "Remember the days of old; consider the years of many generations; ask your father, and he will show you, your elders, and they will tell you." There is no question that our ability to remember is a recurring theme throughout Scripture. Memory is a wonderful ability given to us by God's design. God values memory; so should we, and lament the loss of it.

Memories can be a source of great joy. We take pleasure in remembering the blessings God has given us in the past, and doing so prompts us to thank him and give him glory. Memories motivate us to acts of service and sacrifice in the present. Wisdom often comes as we put several past memories together and learn from them. Memories allow us to see our current lives in sharper perspective. We may be experiencing some times of difficulty, but a memory will come to mind that makes it more tolerable. When we are struggling with doubt about whether we can count on God for help, we need to remember what our Lord did for us on the cross.

Remembering that, we can be confident of his help in our current need. In the Old Testament we see where the prophet Jeremiah, beset by a trying situation, is buoyed by remembering the steadfast love and faithfulness of the Lord:

> Remember my affliction and my wanderings,
> the wormwood and the gall!
> My soul continually remembers it
> and is bowed down within me.
> But this I call to mind,
> and therefore I have hope:
> The steadfast love of the Lord never ceases;
> his mercies never come to an end;
> they are new every morning;
> great is your faithfulness. (Lam. 3:19–23)

God recognizes that we are prone to forget and has prescribed ways to help us remember. He established the Sabbath for a number of reasons, one of which was for the Israelites to remember that they were once slaves in Egypt (Deut. 5:13–15). Annually the Jewish people were commanded to celebrate the Passover to prevent them from forgetting their deliverance from the Egyptians. Through history God commanded various monuments to be made (often a pile of stones) to help his people remember certain events. This practice of prompting our memories was continued in the New Testament when our Lord instituted the Lord's Supper, telling his followers to take the Communion elements "in remembrance of me" (Luke 22:19). Just as God grieves over the many consequences of sin, I suspect he grieves when dementia causes any of his people to forget.

One of the greatest things God ever did to help our poor memories was to give us the Holy Spirit. This is how Jesus described his work: "The Helper, the Holy Spirit, whom the Father will send in my name, he will teach you all things and bring to your remembrance all that I have said to you" (John 14:26). Jesus goes on to describe the peace and the freedom from fear that the reminders from the Holy Spirit will bring to us.

But there are times when it is possible to remember too much. If we remembered every detail of our past experiences, we would be overwhelmed and find it impossible to sort through so much information. In God's providence we forget many potentially distracting details from the past and remember just what we need to make wise choices in the present. Note how Paul was glad to forget some of the past: "One thing I do: forgetting what lies behind and straining forward to what lies ahead, I press on toward the goal for the prize of the upward call of God in Christ Jesus" (Phil. 3:13–14). Paul recognized that if he was to reach the goal of his life in Christ, he needed to forget both the struggles and the glories of the past and press on.

We must recognize that our memories, even at their best, are often poor. I am intrigued that when my wife and I entertain younger couples and ask them to tell us about their first meeting, we often hear two different stories. After the woman relates her cherished memories, the man will chime in and say, "Now let me tell you my version of the story." Further, our memories can be rather fickle and self-serving. How often do we tell a story that shows us off in a little better light than what actually happened? It is not infrequent that what we remember is what we wish had occurred more than what actually did happen. Partly because of our sinful nature, we love to think of ourselves as heroes, portraying ourselves as better than we are.

While we recognize the failure of our memories, one consoling reality is that God has perfect memory. The awesome consequence is that he will never forget us. Most of us take great comfort in this promise:

> Can a woman forget her nursing child,
> > that she should have no compassion on the son of
> > her womb?

> Even these may forget,
>   yet I will not forget you.
> Behold, I have engraved you on the palms of my hands.
>   (Isa. 49:15–16)

We can take comfort in knowing of God's perfect memory, but we can also be consoled that God sometimes chooses to forget. Once we trust Jesus and are born anew, God fully accepts the payment that Jesus made for our sins and removes them from his memory. "I am he who blots out your transgressions for my own sake, and I will not remember your sins" (Isa. 43:25).

Memory and Dementia

Since memory is so important and God values it so highly, we must do whatever we can to preserve the memories of those who have dementia. We can do this by repeatedly telling them the stories of their lives. We should emphasize how God graciously brought them to himself and worked in and through them. And they may never tire of hearing the Bible stories they knew from Sunday school. We need to keep repeating that God loves them and that Jesus died for them. We need to use hymns, either singing or listening, as they will touch their emotional memories.[19] We should also continually remind them of our love for them.

In summary, we can say that as we embrace God's values, they will begin to transform our attitudes toward dementia and allow God to be honored.

Prayer

Heavenly Father, these thoughts convict me, for I also take too much pride in my intellect and in what I have accomplished. I recognize that these do not impress you, for you are so much greater. I know in my heart that my true value lies in the fact that you have made me in your image and have purchased me with the blood of my Savior. Help me to keep that focus. Help me to remember what you want me to remember and to use my memories to gain your wisdom and a spirit of gratitude. I am grateful that you will never forget me even though I may forget you. I pray this for my good and for your honor. Amen.

9

Respect the Dignity of
Those with Dementia

I always looked forward to Jered's appointments at the clinic. Married for sixty-three years, Jered and Jane were deeply in love with each other. Jered suffered from moderately severe dementia, yet he was always pleasant, smiling and congenial. It was beautiful watching the way Jane related to him. When I came into the exam room, she'd be holding his hand and humming a tune while Jered smiled. When I asked him a question, he would nod to Jane, and she would always answer in the plural, not just speaking for herself. He always felt that he was part of the conversation and had some level of input about decisions. In the context of his dementia, Jane clearly respected his God-given dignity. She knew that he was made in the image of God, and she respected him.

Respecting the dignity of a patient with dementia is consistent with biblical values, and it vastly improves the quality of their lives as they deal with this devastating condition. Recently I gave a talk on dementia to a group of seniors. One dear woman sitting in the front row quietly started to cry. I was grateful when she came up to talk at the conclusion of the session. She told me how her husband had recently passed away after several years of dementia. She had never thought about his having dignity through the course of his disease and acknowledged that she had viewed him as a nonperson, a body without a mind. She concluded, "I guess it would have been so much better for both of us had I recognized the dignity of the person he still was."

When we try to respect the dignity of someone with dementia, there are no rules, no cookbook approaches, and every stage of an individual's dementia presents unique challenges to manage. As Christians we must depend on God by his Spirit to help us show respect for our loved ones who have dementia. Still, there are some helpful guidelines we can follow.

Learn from Jesus

We have no record of Jesus interacting with someone afflicted with dementia. Nevertheless, we can learn a lot from him, for he was (and still is!) the great physician who "went about doing good and healing" (Acts 10:38). Jesus dealt with all kinds of physical, mental, and spiritual infirmities. He viewed each individual with compassion, no doubt feeling the tragedy of their disease. Jesus took time with people, spoke to them directly, asked questions, touched them, and selflessly gave of himself. He showed them respect and never blamed them for the afflictions they brought to him. Jesus served even when he was hungry and did not have time to eat. Even physical exhaustion and lack of sleep did not deter him from reaching out to those in need. Jesus helped all kinds of people, from those respected by society to the down and out, from the educated to the unlearned, from the righteous to those trapped in sin. This he did because he loved them, and we can presume he had respect for their dignity, for he created them in the image of God.

One of Jesus's stories that I love is how he healed the blind man Bartimaeus, as recorded in Mark 10. Bartimaeus had been marginalized by his culture. The crowds following Jesus did not believe that Bartimaeus was worth helping, so they tried to silence him when he cried out for help. Jesus, however, stopped and called for him to come to him. Jesus did not treat him as a problem or as a delay in his schedule but took the time to engage him in conversation. He first respected the dignity of Bartimaeus, and then he healed him. What a model for us to follow! But we must take Jesus as our model not only when it is convenient; he has commanded us to do so even when it is inconvenient. When Jesus told the story of a man who had helped a robbery victim in desperate need, he told his listeners to "go, and do likewise" (Luke 10:37). We, too, must show respect for all, including those with dementia. Jesus taught that when we serve those in need, we are actually serving him—a great honor (Matt. 25:40).

Give the Gift of Your Time

God has made us social people; we thrive in the context of relationships. So do many of those with dementia, who are often desperate for human companionship and an escape from loneliness. All too often, they are ignored by others, including those they love. Their loneliness is exacerbated by their illness, for they often quickly forget when someone has spent time with them. I well remember a time when my mother-in-law told my wife that I no longer loved her because I never came to see her. Based on the facts as she viewed them, her conclusion was valid. But the truth was that I had visited her daily, and she had forgotten. Though Mother would forget my visits, the time was not wasted because she enjoyed them at the time.

Contrary to what we might think, the gift of presence is perhaps most significant in the advanced stages of dementia. It is not infrequent at that time for loved ones to feel that their visits do not count for anything. They assume that they won't be recognized or their visit remembered, which may be precisely the wrong conclusion. Those with advanced dementia are often like a three-month-old baby. She will not say, "Mommy, I love you, and I'm so glad you are here," but she is conscious of her mother's presence, allowing her to feel comfortable and secure. Of course, adults with dementia are not children and should never be treated as if they are.

Focus on the Person

When dealing with dementia patients, it is easy to forget that they are unique people with needs, abilities, and potential. We have seen that they still have feelings and need human relationships. We must never see them as a problem to fix. I learned a lot from Elizabeth, a patient I saw several years ago. She came to the office with her sister, Frances. Immediately Frances told me that Elizabeth had wandered out at night, and the police had found her and taken her home. Frances was in tears when she related the incident, fearful that something worse might happen. Elizabeth herself sat there sulking and rather indignantly tried to explain that she had gotten hungry and wanted to go out to get something to eat. Then she said, "But no one listens to me! Aren't I important too?" I was taken aback and ashamed, recognizing that though Frances was telling the truth, Elizabeth deserved to be involved in the discussion, and out of respect for her dignity I should have interrupted Frances and asked Elizabeth what her concerns were at the start of the visit.

All too often, the needs and feelings of people with dementia are discounted. It happens within families as well as in the medical community. How often have I heard remarks like this one: "Mr. Jones was complaining of a headache this afternoon, but he is demented, so who knows what he really feels?" Not only is that bad medicine; it also denies Mr. Jones's value. It focuses on his disease but loses sight of him. Mr. Jones's description of his pain may have been inaccurate, but it should not have been discounted.

Learn How to Communicate

Recognizing people's dignity requires us to aspire to understand what they intend and, as much as possible, assure that they understand us. As we noted earlier, effective communication may require much patience from both speaker and listener. When those with dementia have trouble choosing the right word, they might appreciate a suggestion; at other times, they might find that insulting. A great deal of sensitivity is required in our efforts to respect their dignity. In the later stages of dementia, limited cognition may curtail all verbal communication. At that point various odd behaviors may, in fact, be efforts at communication. Those seeking to understand a specific behavior must be willing to wrestle with what the behavior communicates. Spitting out food might be a way of saying, "I really don't like what you gave me. Could you feed me something else?" Undressing in public may mean, "I want to use the toilet," or "I am too hot." Wandering may mean, "I'm bored and looking for something to do." I hear patients with dementia repeatedly say, "Please let me go home," which frequently means, "Can't I go back to a world where I know and understand what's going on?"

At such times, we can articulate what we think they mean and ask them if we are right. They may be able to answer us. If they spit out food, we can ask if they would rather eat something else. At times they will not be able to respond appropriately. If they are crying out, and we suspect they are trying to tell us about a particular pain, we can ask if they are hurting and, if so, to point to where it hurts. If we fail to recognize that offensive behaviors might actually be efforts at communication, we might get angry. But if we try to correctly interpret their efforts to communicate, we are respecting their dignity.

Effective communication requires not only trying to understand dementia patients but also enabling the patients to understand us. It may help to speak slowly, using short sentences and simple vocabulary and introducing only one thought at a time. Make sure patients have their hearing aids in and glasses on so they can read your lips. Face them when speaking and repeat your words. It may help to use gestures and body language to make sure you get your message across.

Respect Their Autonomy

Remember how Jane responded to my questions to Jered in such a way that she would always include him? In doing so she was showing respect for his autonomy, his desire to have some control over his life. She could have been the big boss and tried to call all the shots, but she consistently deferred to him before making decisions, and though she ultimately made the decisions, he never felt left out. Nobody wants to be told what to do all the time; this is as true of those with dementia as with anyone else.

In earlier stages of dementia, patients are quite capable of making many decisions on their own, and when this is the case their wishes should be followed. As dementia progresses they may still be capable of choosing between a few options but be unable to make wise decisions when faced with more complex issues. So, for example, if you go out for ice cream, offer them a choice between only their two favorite flavors; it is best not to list all the flavors. As decisions become more complex and the implications of those decisions weightier, it is necessary to assess whether patients have the capacity to understand the intricacies of a decision before asking them to make it. A patient quite capable of making a decision about ice cream may not be able to understand the issues involved in deciding to have open-heart surgery. Still, as much as possible, the more we allow the patient to feel they have significant control over their choices, the more we show respect for their inherent dignity.

Respecting autonomy is not always easy. All too often I have seen conflict between an individual with mild to moderate dementia whose primary value is independence, and his family who above everything else desires his safety. I remember Edwardo, who, in the context of a moderate dementia, refused to accept any help from his loving sister and brother-in-law. He insisted on living independently, cooking his own meals, and caring for his apartment. As a result, he lived in filth and became malnourished, and his health rapidly declined. At least his independence did no harm to anyone else. It was extremely troubling not only for his family but also for me, his doctor, to allow him to live that way. Knowing he would be miserable in any other situation, we let him continue till a crisis occurred that required nursing-home care.

Protect Their Dignity

Preserving autonomy as a means of respecting dignity is important, but it is not the only thing to consider. At times we have to protect people with dementia from making mistakes that would discredit their dignity and their reputation. This is necessary because dementia often causes poor judgment, illogical thinking, and lack of inhibition that prevent them from recognizing they have any problem at all. This may be particularly true in frontotemporal degeneration, the form of dementia that Nick and Suzanne had to struggle with. It was complicated because Nick could hold a reasonably decent conversation, and his memory was pretty good.

On first meeting him, no one would guess that he had dementia. Nevertheless, his social skills and judgment were profoundly affected, and his ability to take on a task and get it done (executive function) was very limited. Most distressingly, he lacked the insight to recognize that anything was wrong. Nick insisted that he was capable of continuing in his profession in which many depended on him for their health and livelihood. Everyone but Nick recognized that he was incapable of doing his job. When confronted with his failures, he became upset and angry. Suzanne did not want to embarrass Nick by sharing his diagnosis with his friends and employers. At the same time something had to be done, or others would be hurt and his good reputation damaged. Suzanne finally had to intervene, working behind his back, and she arranged to have Nick relieved of his responsibilities. In this case, respect for autonomy and dignity had to be trumped by the need to protect his good reputation and keep him from hurting others, and in so doing, God was honored.

Driving poses a similar challenge. Allowing those unfit to

continue to drive will not uphold their dignity, and it puts others at risk.

Help Them Find Their Full Potential

I love the title of Rick Phelps's book, *While I Still Can*.[20] Rick, a victim of an early but slowly progressive dementia, was able to write his story in a heartwarming and encouraging way. He did not allow dementia to keep him from helping others find meaning and value. In the midst of his struggle he founded *Memory People*, an Internet support group for dementia sufferers. He became aware of a need and did what he could to meet it.

As much as possible, dementia sufferers should be led to focus on what they are still able to do and not on what they cannot do. When possible we need to do more *with* them and less *to* or *for* them. It may take more time and have its degree of frustration, but it will vastly improve their quality of life. To that end, it is important to seek out opportunities for activities at which they can succeed, and it is equally helpful to steer them away from activities in which they will most likely fail.

Additionally, they can perform regular activities of daily life with their procedural memory, though they may need to be prompted. If you say, "Dad, it's time to get dressed," he may not know where to start, and you might assume he is not capable of doing it on his own. But if you say, "Put on your undershirt first," he may carry on from there; he is not totally dependent. Recognizing his success and giving him exuberant praise also help. As he is dressing you may want to repeatedly keep him focused and encourage him by saying, "Dad, you are doing a great job," or, "I appreciate your doing all these things by yourself—it helps me so much." Such encouragement goes a long way toward allowing patients to feel well, keep functional, and retain dignity.

It is imperative to carefully assess the ability of patients on a day-to-day basis because their capacity to accomplish various tasks will come and go. It is critical to set realistic expectations as well.

Paul admonishes Christians to treat others in a way that is consistent with their abilities: "We urge you, brothers, admonish the idle, encourage the fainthearted, help the weak, be patient with them all" (1 Thess. 5:14). As we exhibit patience, we are to distinguish the idle (the lazy), which is rare in the context of dementia, for most people are trying to do their best, from those who are fainthearted and in need of encouragement and those who are weak (incapable) and need our help. Caregivers do well to match their response to the patient's present mental and physical capacities.

Help Them Find Meaning

When man and woman were created, they were immediately given work to do. God told them to take dominion over the earth, an assignment that provided meaning to their daily lives and made them feel useful. They were not to waste their time or simply amuse themselves. People with dementia may be limited in their ability to accomplish anything of value, but perhaps there are some things they can do. I remember my ninety-year-old grandmother, who suffered from moderately severe dementia, coming to our home once a week to fold the laundry with my mother. It wasn't much, but it allowed her to feel that she was doing something of value.

Meaning, however, does not merely come from what we do. Sometimes it comes simply from who we are and how we feel. We can help people with dementia find meaning by constantly reminding them how much they mean to us and how glad we are to have them around. When they smile, we should tell them how good their smile makes us feel. We can thank them for all they have done for us in the past.

Ray has always been among my favorite patients. He is about my age, a gifted musician and pastor. In his late twenties, several years before I met him, he suffered a cardiac arrest that resulted in severe brain damage. He was unable to remember anything that occurred afterward, though he still remembered events prior to it. In particular he remembered and continued to sing songs he had learned as a child in Sunday school. I was amazed by the repeated testimonies of those who were touched by his singing. Many struggling with a specific issue in their lives would tell how Ray's singing was exactly what they needed to hear. It seems that God used Ray in spite of his dementia to touch a number of needy people deep in their souls. Singing helped Ray find meaning, and he continued to evidence joy in the midst of dementia.

At times our efforts to help someone find meaning can backfire. I heard the story of a distinguished physician I will call Fred Jones, who suffered from severe dementia. He had been an emeritus professor and department chair at a medical school but was now living in a nursing home with other dementia patients. He had spent his whole life serving others, so to honor him, the staff placed his diploma on the wall, put his name, "Dr. Jones," on his door, and respectfully called him "Dr. Jones." But there was a problem. In his desire to find meaning, he wanted to continue to practice medicine and serve his fellow residents. It soon became a crisis, for his field was gynecology, and needless to say, the women living on his floor did not appreciate his services. The staff wisely responded by removing his diploma and changing the nameplate on his door, and they stopped calling him "Dr. Jones." Almost immediately he discontinued his offensive behavior and found meaning in other ways.

Enter Their World

People with more advanced dementia often live in their own little world. This makes it critical for those who relate to them to seek to understand what their world is like. This is intriguingly Christlike, as Jesus took on "the form of a servant, being born in the likeness of men. And being found in human form, he humbled himself" (Phil. 2:7–8). Jesus entered our world so that he could effectively serve us. So, too, we need to enter the world of those who suffer from dementia to effectively serve and respond to them.

Early in the disease, practicing what is termed "reality orientation" can be an effective way to respond to the confusion. When my mom started to think I was someone else, I would gently remind her, "No, Mom, I'm your son, John." Then every time I saw her, I announced myself, saying, "Hi, Mom, it's John." She responded to that for a while, but as her disease progressed, reality orientation was no longer helpful. When later she was convinced I was my dad, my best efforts to tell her otherwise only frustrated her, and she became convinced I was trying to play a trick. That was the time to practice "validation," to enter her world and go along with her thinking. So I responded by telling her how much I loved her and reminiscing about some of the great family times we had in the past. I didn't lie to her, but neither did I correct her, much like entering a child's imaginary world. I remember practicing validation when our eldest son was three. For several weeks he decided he was a frog. Whatever he was eating, he said it was mosquitos. At bedtime he would lie down on his "lily pad," croak, and say, "Ribbit, ribbit," and then go off to sleep. It was great fun, and we never felt obligated to practice "reality orientation" by insisting he wasn't a frog.

There are a number of practical ways in which we can respect dignity by entering the world of people with dementia. Here are a few examples:

1. Get to know their past history, if you are not already familiar with it. Talk to them about stories from their past to allow them to enjoy the memories they still have. It may help to compile a picture book and have them explain the pictures in it.

2. Share some funny stories. They may not understand them, but if you laugh, they may enjoy laughing along with you.

3. Learn what they prefer to be called and use that when speaking with them. It may be the nickname they had as a child.

4. Learn their likes and dislikes from earlier in their lives. You might take them to places they used to enjoy and serve them the comfort foods they once relished. Their forgetfulness may enable you to do this repeatedly. If they used to love mac and cheese, they may be fine eating it every day.

5. Play the music and sing the songs they used to love.

6. Slow down to get into their world. Life for those with dementia moves slowly. Anything you do together will take more time, as it may upset them or even lead to a meltdown if they feel rushed.

7. Respect the constrictions of dementia. As the disease progresses, patients will be less interested in the past and future and more focused on the present. They will be less interested in news of the world outside and may not want to leave the comfort of their home or room. What is going on in the lives of other people may not be important to them; eventually, however, they will care only about how they feel in the here and now. To respect their dignity, those around them must learn to enjoy the present moment with them. At times, being touched and held may be all they want. Recognize that caregivers' need for activity may be far greater than theirs.

8. Respect their resistance to change. Establish routines they are comfortable with. Having meals at the same time and going to bed and getting up on a regular schedule are usually best. The world they live in does not require much variety.

9. If they perceive that you did something wrong and have become upset by it, accept that their understanding of what happened may be totally different from yours. Do not make excuses but apologize profusely. That will affirm them, avoid arguments, and allow them to feel better.

Prayer

Heavenly Father, respecting the dignity of others gets very complicated, and I have a lot to learn. Grant me the wisdom and creativity I need to follow the example of Jesus and serve others as he would. Transform my view of those with dementia and allow me to see Jesus in them and treat them with the same dignity that I would see in my Savior. I pray this for my good, the good of those I know with dementia, and for your honor. Amen.

10

Meet the Needs of Those
with Dementia

To say that people with dementia are needy people is a gross understatement. The challenge of dealing with their needs is greatly increased when the caregiver does not know what those needs are. Even patients themselves may fail to understand what they need; they just know they are uncomfortable and unable to communicate it to others. Discovering these needs requires the same type of detective work as figuring out how to comfort a crying three-month-old whose parents must discern whether she needs to be held, changed, or fed or is in pain. At the clinic, many patients with dementia simply say they feel lousy. When I ask them for more words, they often say, "You know, I just feel lousy." Such vague complaints make my job as a physician really tough; it requires a lot of time and probing. Is the source of the complaint physical, emotional, or spiritual? Or is it a combination of all three? Though difficult, it is worth my while to rise to the challenge and do everything I can to help, for this is one way in which God is honored through dementia.

Denise could be at her wits' end when frustrated with Dave.

One time she brought him to the office and told me that for several days he had been groaning and saying, "I don't feel well; I just don't feel well. Please help me." On the first day he pointed to his stomach, but later it was his head, and at other times he would just cry. He had no fever and was eating well, his plumbing was working, and he did not appear to be in pain. There was no obvious diagnosis, but, thankfully, we looked at his urine and found a urinary tract infection, which we were able to treat. On another occasion he came in with much the same confusing picture, but we found nothing. Thankfully, two days later the symptoms, whatever they were, disappeared. At another time, he could not stop talking about his brother who had died at age ten, and Dave appeared to be depressed. He felt better after a change in his antidepressant. No matter how he felt, Denise tried to understand his need, and if she couldn't figure out what was troubling him, she brought him to see me. She never wanted to overlook any treatable cause of his distress, but it was difficult to advise her as to when she should bring him in and when it was safe to just watch. My best advice was not so much to listen to Dave but to look at him. If he looked like he was in distress, he needed to see me, even if he denied problems. Similarly, if he was complaining of something but looked healthy, it could be observed safely at home. If she exhausted all efforts to understand the source of his problem with no success, she would sit and hold him, and they would cry together. Then she would pray with him. What impressed me was the steadfastness of her love in spite of her frustration and the multiple ways in which she sought to make him feel better.

Attend to Their Physical Needs

Let's think some about physical needs. First, we must remember that people with dementia get sick and develop chronic diseases just like anyone else. Their arthritis hurts when they walk too far. They may not be able to tell you; instead, they may simply refuse to keep going. Whatever the case, their problems should not be ignored. They may demonstrate shortness of breath with various activities. When they have such symptoms, they should be taken to the doctor for proper diagnosis and treatment. The presence of dementia never justifies ignoring basic physical needs.

Just like the rest of us, dementia patients need the basic comforts in life. They get hot in the heat and cold in the cold. Because they might not be able to communicate their discomfort, experience and sensitivity are required by caregivers.

People with dementia will benefit from exercise. Getting out for walks helps to loosen up muscles, control weight, improve the quality of sleep, and ward off depression. Helping patients maintain good muscle strength and control their weight has the added advantage that when they enter the later stages of dementia and become more dependent, they will be easier to care for.

Additionally, they still have food preferences. This will include not only the taste but also the texture of their food. Chewing problems are common. There will be certain foods that they want all the time, and since they don't remember what they had yesterday, it is okay to give them the same food day after day. When patients are no longer able to feed themselves, the human contact that occurs from being fed may become a daily high point. Others will lose their appetite, and if that happens they may benefit from daily supplements such as Ensure. Good, balanced nutrition is always beneficial but not something to fight about.

Many persons with dementia still care how they look. Ladies may want to have their hair done regularly, use their makeup, and dress in an attractive style (though they may prefer the style and even the clothes they wore thirty years ago). Men will want to be shaved and may want to wear the jackets and ties they used to wear to the office if that was their custom. People with dementia appreciate compliments about how good they look. Incidentally, they may also appreciate the way their family and friends appear in their presence. One way we can honor people is by dressing nicely for them.

Dementia does not alter our ability to experience pleasure. Victims of dementia may enjoy pleasing aromas and be put off by offensive ones. They may like good music and admire pretty scenes or pictures. I have seen people with dementia sit and look at a picture for long periods, occasionally making a comment about something that strikes them. They will often enjoy human touch. They may want their loved ones to hold their hands or put an arm around them; back or neck rubs may become the thrill of the day. A kiss may be appreciated.

Attend to Their Social Needs

We have seen that people with dementia continue to be social beings. We have discussed how one of the greatest gifts is presence, simply spending time with them. But their social needs may go beyond contact with caregivers and closest family. Even then, they may be rather particular about who they spend time with. In addition, while they may be okay in one-on-one situations, they may not do well in large groups. At a large, noisy family gathering, they may become confused and irritable, possibly leading to a meltdown. They may do better in a room by themselves with just one other person. A break between social visits may also help.

Like the rest of us, those with dementia do not like to be talked about, embarrassed, or corrected in public. There are times when it may be necessary to explain to others that the patient has memory problems, but this needs to be done discreetly. In the same way, they don't want their mistakes and inadequacies pointed out—an important issue to keep in mind, since those with dementia tend to make a lot of mistakes. When possible, it's more fitting to come alongside and help them avoid a mistake. If this is not possible, it is wise not to correct them but rather to overlook their blunder. Should there be likelihood of the problem reccurring, it is wise to keep the patient out of that situation. Remember that the very nature of dementia makes learning very difficult. When dealing with my mother in her dementia, I quickly learned that she would not be able to answer when I asked her what she'd done that day. She would get frustrated when she couldn't tell me. It was fine, though, to ask her if she'd enjoyed the day. None of us likes our ignorance to show. Just as we get frustrated by dementia sufferers repeatedly asking questions we have already answered, we do not want to frustrate them by asking questions they cannot answer.

Before we leave the topic of how we can help with social needs, I need to mention that one of the most difficult social situations I have faced is when two people with dementia want to have a sexual relationship. This is particularly problematic for Christians who have honored their Lord by living chaste and godly lives, with or without a spouse. I believe that we should honor their previous chastity and do everything possible to prevent them from doing anything they wouldn't have done prior to dementia. At times this requires enforced physical separation and at other times use of an antidepressant, sedative, or hormonal manipulation to quell the sexual drives.

Attend to Their Emotional Needs

We have seen earlier both that God values emotions and that persons with dementia still have emotions. We must never allow their cognitive impairment to blind us to their emotional needs. They may *feel* much more than they *know*, and how they *feel* may be far more important to them than what they *know*. People with dementia want to be loved, and they want to love others. How love is expressed to someone with dementia will change as the disease progresses. Early on it may be conveyed by doing things together or giving them gifts (my preference would be homemade chocolate desserts). As the dementia progresses, love may be conveyed by repeating phrases such as "I love you." Smiles and affectionate pats on the back may help convince them of your love. The fact is, loved ones can never express their love too much. Our love was founded on the relationship we had with them before the onset of dementia, but though it may be more difficult, we must learn to love them as they are today. We must also recognize that loving someone with dementia will likely not be a sentimental, romanticized love but one that more closely fits the biblical norm of a serving, self-sacrificing love patterned on Jesus's love for us.

In addition to love, a person with dementia needs to experience other positive emotions. These include joy and happiness. When possible they need to laugh. They also need to be thankful. We need to sit and review with them many of the good things in life and help them appreciate more of God's goodness while giving thanks to him. Another positive emotion they can experience is contentment. This may not be at all easy in the early and middle stages of dementia, when they are still conscious of their disabilities, but it may show up in the later stages, when many do show a high level of contentment.

There may be times when the emotions of anger, fear, or sadness predominate. These emotions can be magnified by a lack of inhibition and lead to full-blown loss of control, or meltdowns. In these situations a good caregiver will learn to recognize the first signs of a meltdown and attempt to distract the patient before it escalates. The underlying anger or frustration may blow over and be forgotten, but, if not, it is necessary to somehow direct patients to disperse the negativity. It may be possible to talk them through it, go out for a vigorous walk, or simply engage in some other activity to distract them.

Attend to Their Spiritual Needs

The relationship between mind and spirit is fascinating yet poorly understood. Scripture is clear that all human beings are essentially a union of body and soul. Our minds have thoughts, wills, and emotions, none of which can be adequately explained on the basis of our physical brains. Though modern science uses functional MRIs to locate areas of the brain associated with emotions and thoughts, this does not mean that our physical brains are their only source. We must also understand that within our minds, we have a spiritual awareness, including a consciousness of God (Rom. 1:20).

The apostle Paul typically used the terms *soul* and *spirit* interchangeably and thus saw them as equivalents, but in one passage he notes a distinction between mind and spirit: "What am I to do? I will pray with my spirit, but I will pray with my mind also; I will sing praise with my spirit, but I will sing with my mind also" (1 Cor. 14:15). Just like any other areas of our brains, the part where spiritual activity is located can be damaged by dementia; even so we have no reason to assume that the Spirit of God cannot still work in the soul of someone with dementia. We know that through the early and mid-stages, patients can have active and vibrant spiritual lives, though perhaps not to the degree enjoyed before the illness struck. In the later stages, we have no clear idea of what goes on in their spirits, but we have no evidence that the Holy Spirit does not continue to relate to them as their comforter and continue to mold their characters. Theologian Stephen Sapp writes:

> Furthermore, what evidence really exists that God does *not* still come to those who are cognitively impaired? The widely held assumption that a person's capacity to relate to God is lost when he or she loses cognitive function may just sell God short. . . . God can still relate to a person even if his or her ability to relate to God (or to other people) appears lost.[21]

With the basic assumption that God, by his Spirit, continues to work in the lives of those at all stages of dementia, we ask how we can be part of that process. There are many ways, but let's consider just a few.

Remind them that God has not forgotten them. God's love for us does not depend on our response to him. Though we may forget him, he will never forget us. How comforting for all of us to know that "if we are faithless, he remains faithful" (2 Tim. 2:13).

Talk about the Lord. Psychologist Benjamin Mast has written

Second Forgetting: Remembering the Power of the Gospel during Alzheimer's Disease.[22] This insightful book is based on extensive experience demonstrating that talking about the Lord, his love, and the good news of the gospel through the course of everyday life can slowly set the tone for the thinking of one suffering from dementia and become part of their lasting spiritual memories. It is somewhat reminiscent of how parents in Israel were to raise their children:

> These words that I command you today shall be on your heart. You shall teach them diligently to your children, and shall talk of them when you sit in your house, and when you walk by the way, and when you lie down, and when you rise. You shall bind them as a sign on your hand, and they shall be as frontlets between your eyes. You shall write them on the doorposts of your house and on your gates. (Deut. 6:6–9)

All Christians should spend a lot of time talking about the Lord; the more we learn to concentrate our attention on him, the better prepared we will be should dementia strike. If we have not been living with an emphasis on the Lord, the sooner we begin, the more helpful it will be as dementia progresses.

Focus on the cross. The sooner we turn the focus to the cross, the better, but it is never too late to do so. We need to keep talking with patients about the cross and what Jesus endured for us. Many Christians are not big on using visual cues to remind people of the cross, but such cues can be useful for dementia patients. Pictures may communicate more effectively than words. Though it is not a part of my tradition, I have seen some people with severe dementia blessed by being able to hold a cross and focus on it. If your church approves, one practice I have found meaningful is to share communion with dementia sufferers who can no longer attend worship services. If they have been in the regular practice of remembering our Lord's death in the broken bread and the cup, these elements may trigger precious emotional and procedural memories.

Focus on heaven. We need to be frequently reminded that our eternal future with God in heaven will be truly glorious. The victims of dementia, like us, need to continually hear the hope of resurrection and the eternal life we look forward to. We may not know much about heaven, but what we do know is worth reflection. Paul writes, "What no eye has seen, nor ear heard, nor the heart of man imagined, what God has prepared for those who love him" (1 Cor. 2:9). What a beautiful picture we see: "Behold, the dwelling place of God is with man. He will dwell with them, and they will be his people, and God himself will be with them as their God. He will wipe away every tear from their eyes, and death shall be no more, neither shall there be mourning, nor crying, nor pain anymore, for the former things have passed away" (Rev. 21:3–4). How reassuring that one of those former things is dementia—it will have passed away. As much as possible, people suffering from dementia should be reminded of their eternal hope.

Use Scripture. The further dementia progresses, the less cognitive material sufferers can handle at any one time. Early in their disease it may be appropriate to read aloud an entire passage and then discuss it with them. As dementia progresses, it may be one verse at a time. Reading a passage that the patient was once familiar with or, better yet, had memorized is most effective. Make sure you read it in the same translation that they memorized years before. One little game I played with my dad as his dementia was getting worse was to quote the beginning of a verse and then let him finish it. He may not have been able to tell me what had happened that morning, but when I said, "For God so . . . ," Dad would quickly pick it up and say, ". . . loved the world, that he gave his only begotten son, that whosoever believeth in him should not perish, but have everlasting life" (John 3:16 KJV). Then he would sigh, sit back, and smile. He could do that with any number of verses.

Robert Davis, the pastor who wrote of his own experience of

dementia, spoke of the comfort he received when his wife recorded long passages of Scripture that he could listen to when he was unable to sleep. He found the comfort of God's Word, combined with hearing a familiar voice, soothing and comforting.

Pray together. Many Christians are great prayer warriors throughout their lives. They have cultivated a deep relationship with God and love to spend time in his presence, not just asking him for things but worshiping him, thanking him, and confessing their sin. Even with dementia, they can still do this. Though it is important for others to pray for those with dementia, it is equally important to pray with them. For many mature believers, prayer has become part of their procedural memory, and they are able to pray aloud with amazing clarity. We should also be mindful that even when they cannot clearly articulate their prayers, we have our Lord's promise: "Likewise the Spirit helps us in our weakness. For we do not know what to pray for as we ought, but the Spirit himself intercedes for us with groanings too deep for words. And he who searches hearts knows what is the mind of the Spirit, because the Spirit intercedes for the saints according to the will of God" (Rom. 8:26–27). In the mid- to later stages of my mother's dementia, when it was difficult to have a conversation with her, I would ask her if we could pray together over the phone. Unable to lead in prayer, she appreciated when I would pray for each one in the family. She wanted to continue her long-standing practice of praying for her children and grandchildren though unable to do so on her own.

Use hymns they know. Music is a wonderful way to reach the spirit of people with dementia. Our church used to offer a worship service in the assisted-living facility next door. One dear friend was there every weekend playing his guitar and singing the old hymns. We were amazed how many of the residents, even with dementia, would either sing along or sit smiling in quiet reverie. I would on occasion be asked to present a brief devotional. In spite of my best efforts, many slept or did not follow even the simplest of thoughts. It was not the preaching that reached their souls; it was the music.

My mother loved to sing. She enjoyed hymns and many other genres of music. We were impressed that even in her more advanced dementia she still knew the words and music often better than we did. During the last year of her life, I put together thirty minutes of hymns on a little MP3 player that could be clipped to her dress. If it was set to "shuffle" and "repeat," she could listen to it all day. The nurses told me she was calmed by the music and took pleasure in it. It made no difference that she listened to the same songs over and over, for though she forgot what they were, she enjoyed the present moment.

Encourage them to serve. Though dementia will progressively reduce its victims' ability to do things for others, they will still be able to serve during the early stages of the disease. One of the challenges of being a good caregiver is to find ways for the patient to serve others consistent with their present abilities. Doing little things that seem insignificant may help those with dementia find meaning and contentment, especially when accompanied by words of deep appreciation. If able, they may do some simple cleaning around the house or even at church. I have seen some with dementia greet people at church while handing out bulletins. The opportunities are numerous and limited only by the individual's ability and the caregiver's energy and creativity.

Deal with Difficult Spiritual Situations

Dementia can negatively transform the personalities of some of the godliest saints, which can be extremely distressing for caretakers who may at times despair of patients' very salvation and wonder if they are actually in the presence of a demon. Caregivers have to deal with patients' swearing, profanity, and sexual references, all of which were unimaginable in former years. There is no simple answer, and it is essential to recognize that these negative changes are caused by the disease. The difference between the experience of those with dementia and those without may not be the presence of bad thoughts but rather the inability to restrain them. All of us, when functioning with normal brains, entertain occasional nasty, sinful thoughts. By God's grace and with the help of his Spirit we suppress them and avoid saying them publicly. With the lack of inhibition associated with dementia, the opposite can be the case, and a lot of unsavory thoughts spill out.

As Mother's dementia progressed and her whole personality changed, allowing her to do and say inappropriate things to others, I was conscious of Job's request that the Lord would cut him off before he "denied the words of the Holy One" (Job 6:10). One of my prayers for Mother was that the Lord would take her home before she said or did things that would have embarrassed her and contradicted her deep love for and trust in the Lord.

Yet I do not believe we can be totally superficial and reassuring in such situations. We know that Satan is active in this world and that he still "prowls around like a roaring lion, seeking someone to devour" (1 Pet. 5:8). Satanic influence in the context of dementia may be unusual but is not impossible. If you have serious questions about it, seek help from discerning spiritual leaders.

As I did, you too will benefit from the testimony of two men who were suffering from dementia. First is that of Rick Phelps: "First and foremost I need to thank God. My struggle with this disease has brought me to a closer relationship with Him."[23] The other is from pastor Robert Davis: "The result of this experience was not commitment to a blind resignation, but a recommitment to a loving Father who had called me, molded me, healed me, and empowered me for his service."[24] Dementia does not close the door to an experience with God.

Exploring and lovingly seeking to meet the many needs of those with dementia is a wonderful way to see God honored through the experience.

Prayer

Heavenly Father, as I consider all the needs that dementia presents, it is overwhelming. I feel so inadequate. I know I am weak, but you are strong. Grant me the love, strength, insight, discernment, and wisdom to provide for the needs that confront me. I pray this for my own good and for your honor. Amen.

11

What Should the Church Do?

I never cease to be amazed at how God views his church. When I look at the church I see a group of sinners who sincerely desire to honor God in their worship, have their characters transformed, and love each other; but all too often we fail to do so. Yet God sees the church as "his body, the fullness of him who fills all in all" (Eph. 1:23). Living up to how God views his church is a tall order, to say the least. God designed the church to reflect all he is in his love, wisdom, and power. As God is involved in the world, so should his church be. For our specific purpose, as God loves and cares for those with dementia, so should his church.

Dave and Denise had been active in their local congregation all of their adult lives. They had each served in a variety of capacities, and most of their close friends were from their church. One day I was talking to Denise about caring for Dave, and she told me how much she appreciated the support her church had been giving. She mentioned that they were faithfully praying for both her and Dave, and she especially appreciated the phone calls and visits from the pastoral staff and their many friends. She said, "It's so nice when they take the time to come over and pray with us. It tells me that even though Dave may seem to have forgotten them, they have not forgotten us, and it assures me that God has not forgotten us either." Denise experienced some of the ways in which a church can bless victims of dementia and their families.

Christian psychologist Benjamin Mast claims, "A community formed by the gospel has the potential to transform Alzheimer's care."[25] Perhaps that is one way in which the church as the body of Christ can actually be the fullness of God. This leads us to consider *how* the church should be involved. There are a number of ways.

Establish Christians Firmly in the Practices of Their Faith

The best thing that a local church can do to prepare victims and caregivers for the spiritual challenges of dementia is to instill in them a deep and joyful experience with Jesus. If Christians memorize Scripture and sing hymns often enough to ingrain them in their brains, they may become part of their emotional and procedural memories, thereby being more likely to recall them once faced with dementia. For the caregiver, Scripture and hymns may sustain them through days of challenge and difficulty when they have so little time to nurture their own spiritual lives.

Dr. Mast emphasizes this when he writes, "Even in a locked memory care unit of a nursing home, [many] seem as if they are completely unaware of what is going on. But when they hear an old hymn that they know and love, they light up and sing every word of it. It is a beautiful picture of how they have this hymn, this truth, embedded deep within them, and they can access it when they are prompted."[26] There is no guarantee that prayer, reading the Scriptures, and other disciplines of the Christian life established prior to the onset of dementia will continue through the course of the disease, but it is fairly certain that if they were not practiced before the onset of dementia, they will not be practiced afterward.

Proactively Teach a Theology of Suffering

The church loves to celebrate God's love and goodness, and well she should. God has richly blessed us not only with salvation but with so many of the other good things he pours into our lives. As we experience more of God's love, we should love him more in return. When our Lord was asked to define the greatest commandment, he responded, "You shall love the Lord your God with all your heart and with all your soul and with all your mind. This is the great and first commandment. And a second is like it: You shall love your neighbor as yourself" (Matt. 22:37–39). In practice this means that our love for God and others should supersede our love for our own comfort and pleasure. Loving God and neighbor with all our hearts, souls, and minds is excellent preparation for dealing with dementia.

As we celebrate God's goodness, we must recognize that part of his loving care for us is allowing difficulties to come into our lives—such as dementia. We cannot deny that dealing with dementia, whether from the perspective of the patient, the caregiver, or other observers, involves emotional, spiritual, and at times even physical suffering. To handle it well, Christians need to be taught early in their lives that God is in control, that he always does what is good, and that we can trust him through the hard times of life. If we are going to endure suffering in a way that honors God, we need a robust understanding of how God uses suffering. This must start with an understanding of who God is.

God is all powerful, loving, sovereign, and eternal. I come back to one of my favorite Bible verses: "One thing God has spoken, two things I have heard: 'Power belongs to you, God, and with you, Lord, is unfailing love'" (Ps. 62:11–12 NIV). When we experience even the most difficult trials in life, we can still affirm that God is both strong and loving. Dementia does not take God by surprise. Elsewhere the psalmist affirms: "Our God is in the heavens; he does all that he pleases" (Ps. 115:3). Another reassuring characteristic of God is that while we are moving through time and experiencing one event after another in sequence, God is always present. Moses writes in his psalm, "From everlasting to everlasting you are God" (Ps. 90:2). That means that while we are enduring the process, God sees the end result. In that, we can be most comforted. In a very real sense God already sees us in heaven, enjoying his presence, with our suffering all past. From that point of view, the trial of dementia may actually seem rather trivial.

I can never think about going through the difficulties of life without looking at an etching that sits over my desk. It is a picture of a potter leaning over his wheel shaping a piece of clay. Underneath are God's words spoken through the prophet Jeremiah: "Behold, like the clay in the potter's hand, so are you in my hand" (Jer. 18:6). What a beautiful picture. But then I have to ask if I would volunteer to be plopped down on a wheel, spun around at 500 rpms, and have all my rough edges knocked off. Who, though, would I trust more to be the potter than my loving heavenly Father? Dementia, like the potter's wheel, is a tool God uses to shape character.

Suffering is God's will for us. God's people must understand that suffering is not a tragic mistake that comes into our lives. Scripture assures us that it is the norm for a Christian. In the book of Acts the apostles taught that "through many tribulations we must enter the kingdom of God" (Acts 14:22). Peter writes, "Let those who suffer according to God's will entrust their souls to a faithful Creator" (1 Pet. 4:19). Yes, times of suffering are not a tragic mistake in God's universe; he ordains them according to his will.

Suffering has purpose. We can be assured that whatever happens, God has a purpose for it. Elsewhere the psalmist affirms that God's purpose goes along with his love for us: "The LORD will fulfill his purpose for me; your steadfast love, O LORD, endures forever" (Ps. 138:8). We get another glimpse into God's control over all things, good and bad, in this rather striking verse from Proverbs, "The LORD has made everything for its purpose, even the wicked for the day of trouble" (Prov. 16:4). God's purposes in dementia include the patient, the caregiver, those in the church, and members of the larger community; in God's omniscience everyone involved will in some way and at some time benefit from it. Theologian John Swinton writes:

> Not to suggest that God is indifferent to the suffering that dementia brings. It is, however, to emphasize that dementia has meaning. It is not punishment; it is not the work of the devil. It is a mystery which is firmly rooted in God's creative and redemptive actions in and for the world. It may not be understandable. It may make us angry, distressed, even outraged. But it is not without meaning. In this sense, people with dementia are part of the flux of fallen humanity, but their condition does not alter their meaningfulness and their lovableness.[27]

Believers need to focus on the cross rather than on their circumstances. Jesus did not call us to a life of comfort and pleasure. Whoever follows him, he said, must "deny himself and take up his cross and follow me" (Mark 8:34). We err when we allow the circumstances of our lives to be the measure of God's love rather than looking at the cross of Jesus and seeing the vastness of God's love demonstrated there. When we focus on the cross, we see the trials of dementia in a totally different light. We may feel it is unfair that we have to endure its effects, but, needless to say, the cruel death that Jesus experienced for us was not fair either. Pastor Timothy Keller expresses this beautifully:

> But then, there you are at the cross with the few of his disciples who have the stomach to watch. And you hear people say, "I've had it with this God. How could he abandon the best man we have ever seen? *I don't see how God could bring any good out of this.*" What would you say? You would likely agree. And yet you are standing there looking at the greatest, most brilliant thing God could ever do for the human race. On the cross, both justice and love are being satisfied—evil, sin and death are being defeated. You are looking at an absolute beauty, but because you cannot fit it into your own limited understanding, you are in danger of walking away from God.[28]

Suffering can be counted a privilege for a Christian. At first it may be hard to consider suffering as a privilege, especially when it is caused by dementia, but when we consider what Jesus endured for us and some of the good results that God can accomplish through dementia, we may actually count it so. Paul writes, "It has been granted to you that for the sake of Christ you should not only believe in him but also suffer for his sake" (Phil. 1:29).

Suffering and glory are often linked. Suffering is repeatedly associated with glory in the New Testament. Consider these passages:

> Was it not necessary that the Christ should suffer these things and enter into his glory? (Luke 24:26)

> I consider that the sufferings of this present time are not worth comparing with the glory that is to be revealed to us. (Rom. 8:18)

> We see him who for a little while was made lower than the angels, namely Jesus, crowned with glory and honor because of the suffering of death, so that by the grace of God he might taste death for everyone. For it was fitting that he, for whom and by whom all things exist, in bringing many sons to glory, should make the founder of their salvation perfect through suffering. (Heb. 2:9–10)

> After you have suffered a little while, the God of all grace, who has called you to his eternal glory in Christ, will himself restore, confirm, strengthen, and establish you. (1 Pet. 5:10)

We may not always (or even frequently) understand how the suffering associated with dementia uniquely prepares us for the glory of God's presence, especially while enduring it. But if we know our Bibles and have been taught a biblical view of suffering, we will be better prepared when we experience it. I have heard a few (not many) wonderful sermons over the years on the role of suffering in the Christian life, but I don't recall hearing the word *dementia* ever mentioned. For a disease that is likely to affect one-third of those in the congregation, it seems to me that the church is failing to address this issue. We need to do a better job equipping God's people to cope with the suffering associated with dementia.

Teach What It Means to Be Fully Human

In a day when there is much confusion as to what it means to be a person, the church must teach a robust view of personhood that is based on our being made in the image of God, as we saw earlier. Most church members would affirm that all people are made in God's image, but if asked what that really means, it's likely they would say something like, "Well, I guess that means they are like God, they are intelligent, can make their own choices, and have the ability to relate to others." If you probed further and asked, "Does that mean people with severe dementia, who are not intelligent, cannot make their own choices, and do not have the ability to relate to others, no longer reflect God's image?" They would likely look surprised, perhaps a bit uncomfortable, and say, "I'm not sure." If we pursued our pretend discussion one step further and asked, "Does that mean they are not persons?" the answer hopefully would be, "I didn't mean that." Just as I never recall hearing the word *dementia* in a sermon, I do not recall being taught in church that personhood is an ontological (something that is true by definition) state and that all those made in God's image are persons possessed with inherent dignity and worthy of the respect we would give to the one whose image they bear.

Whether we are willing to face these difficult questions or not, we have to acknowledge that they are important, and the consequences of our taking the wrong view can be devastating. The only way to prevent such tragic errors is for the church to make a priority of teaching that all humans are persons made in the image of God and should therefore be treated with respect for the dignity they possess. If we all saw the victims of dementia as fully human persons made in God's image, it would profoundly impact the way the church responds to them.

Develop a Culture of Caring and Serving

Jesus taught that one of the hallmarks of his followers should be the love they share with one another. "By this all people will know that you are my disciples, if you have love for one another" (John 13:35). More forcefully Paul says, "Bear one another's burdens, and so fulfill the law of Christ" (Gal. 6:2). Local churches need to teach the importance of and then provide opportunities for its members to be actively involved in the lives of needy congregants. Care must not be solely the role of the deacons or the benevolence fund; everyone in the church is called to recognize needs and be ready to provide practical help.

In our present context the church needs to appreciate that it is a privilege to serve those with dementia. The state may provide some care, as may their friends and family members, but the church is honored to share in the work. And from an individual standpoint, those who aid in caring for dementia sufferers are better prepared to handle the circumstances should they one day hit close to home.

Provide Spiritually for Those with Dementia

Each case of dementia has unique aspects, so no single approach is best for all. Yet in every case, patients and their caregivers must be made to feel welcome at church, even when their presence may cause some uncomfortable moments. Offering hugs and words of appreciation will make them feel welcome. When it comes to meeting spiritual needs, the church has a number of responsibilities

Recognize the dementia sufferer's need for worship. God wants his people to gather together with other believers. His command that believers not neglect meeting together (Heb. 10:25) tells us of its importance and is all inclusive. Yet those with dementia may no longer benefit from attending large services. The large group size can be intimidating, loud noises disturbing, and rapidly paced activities hard to follow. The experience may provoke extreme confusion, possibly a meltdown. Church leaders should be aware of this prospect and provide alternatives, such as seating in an overflow room. Some churches are equipped to provide special worship services for attendees with dementia. I know of several large churches that hold such services, which include lots of singing, shorter sermons, and a warm, welcoming atmosphere. Since these programs are labor intensive, they can be done only with the commitment of a large group. But even with the best programming, those with cognitive impairment will eventually be unable to attend any type of worship service. When that time comes, worshiping in a small-group context may be an option. These smaller, more intimate gatherings are able to serve the needs of dementia sufferers. However, even this type of fellowship will become prohibitive over time, which is why it is critical that even though they may forget the church, the church must not forget them.

Visitation. The lay leadership and the pastoral team should have a regular schedule for home visits as well as visits to assisted-living and nursing homes. This becomes especially important once dementia patients can no longer attend services. Because dementia breeds loneliness for both patients and caregivers, a visit from the church can provide welcome relief. Even if the patient is quick to forget the visits, they will no doubt be enjoyed at the time. A visit provides the opportunity to read Scripture, pray, and converse to the extent that the patient and caregiver are able.

When dementia became a personal issue for pastor Robert Davis, his view on how to conduct pastoral visits changed. He wrote that instead of bringing patients CDs of messages, he would sit and slowly read a familiar passage of Scripture, a poem, or a hymn. Reminding patients of their former contributions to the church body is also encouraging. Practically, these visits allow church leadership to monitor how things are going in the patient's home and to discover if other assistance is needed.

Help them find a place to serve. Dementia sufferers may be incapable of serving as they have done in times past, but there are other things they can do. Though unable to teach a class, they might be able to arrange chairs in the classroom. When the church takes time to consider the abilities of those with dementia and monitor them over time, providing ways for them to serve accordingly, God is honored.

Prayer. Those with dementia and their caregivers should remain on the church's prayer list and be prayed for during the regular service. The church should pray for their healing and for perseverance, asking also that God be honored throughout the illness. Those with dementia can pray as well. I have been amazed at the coherent prayers of some of my patients. When appropriate it is wise to give them the opportunity to lead the congregation in prayer.

Support groups. Early in the course of dementia, patients may benefit from getting together with those in a similar situation. Often there is an insufficient number of dementia sufferers within a single congregation from which to form a dedicated group, but several congregations, particularly in urban areas, can cooperate to sponsor one.

Care for Caregivers

The church can have an even greater impact on caregivers than on dementia sufferers.

Commissioning. Allow me to share with you one of my dreams: picture a local church taking time to commission a caregiver to the ministry to which God has called them. We commission our missionaries, our pastors, and our Sunday school teachers. How about our caregivers?

Welcoming and accepting. Efforts must be made to allow caregivers to get to church as often as possible. This may require a willingness of some from the congregation to forgo attending, themselves, in order to stay with the dementia patient.

Pastoral visits. Ostensibly, pastoral visits are intended to encourage dementia patients, but those who receive the greatest benefit are often the caregivers. With today's technologies, people do not need to go to church to hear good music and wonderful sermons or to share in confession or prayer, but what they can never get elsewhere is the personal concern and presence of a pastor and fellow Christians.

Providing respite and help at home. Early in the course of dementia a caregiver should meet with those in the local church, possibly the deacons or other help ministries, and begin to talk about ways the church can be involved as the patient's dementia progresses. A critical turning point for caregivers occurs when the patient's disease progresses to the point where the patient cannot be left alone. At that time the practical needs of caregivers dramatically increase. They may need help with housecleaning, yard work, and getting out of the house to shop and just unwind. If several people from the church wish to provide in-home support, it may be wise for the church to offer some training beforehand.

Prayer support. We have mentioned the value of remembering caregivers in corporate prayer, but perhaps equally important are one-to-one prayer sessions. Praying with a caregiver is best done in person, but when that is impossible, praying over the phone is an option. The prayers offered should not be for the caregiver only; the caregiver should be given the chance to pray for others as well, which will do wonders for the caregiver's spirit.

Counsel. Caregivers frequently need a listening ear for and wise counsel about the challenges they face. Counsel may come from a pastor, a counselor on the church staff, or a layperson who has some experience with the unique challenges of dementia.

Maintaining a file of community services. A practical way the church can help is to link caregivers to applicable services in the community. Significant time and effort are required to research the help they need, so a great burden is lifted if someone from the church will take time to compile a list of community resources.

Family mediation. Dementia care often disrupts family unity, especially when the care is disproportionately carried by one person. Sensitive church leadership should recognize signs of disharmony and volunteer to intervene when necessary. This is imperative when the entire family worships within the congregation.

Financial help. Some caregivers must forgo employment to care for a dementia patient, and mounting expenses quickly drain available resources. Adult day care, in-home professional help, special equipment, a hospital bed, house adaptations such as grab bars or ramps, special foods, and ultimately the cost of a nursing home quickly add up. Scripture requires the church to provide for widows whose families cannot do so. Should they not also help with the financial burden of caring for someone with dementia?

Providing transportation. This practical need can be met by almost anyone with a car. The caregiver has to focus on the patient and is therefore often unable to drive. A driver need not know anything about dementia or even the patient to provide this crucial service.

Support groups. A support group can begin simply by connecting caregivers who are members of the same church. Ideally, such a group will consist of both those relatively new to caregiving and those with more experience. The group may develop into a more formal ministry as more people get involved. If a church has a professional in the congregation, perhaps a nurse or a physician with experience in dementia care, he or she may be able to lead the ministry.

The key question we are exploring is how God can be honored in the midst of dementia. Having the church involved is an essential part of the answer. Jesus said, "Let your light shine before others, so that they may see your good works and give glory to your Father who is in heaven" (Matt. 5:16). The apostle John says, "No one has ever seen God; if we love one another, God abides in us and his love is perfected in us" (1 John 4:12). Though the world around us has never seen God, they may get a glimpse into what his love is like by observing the way we as his church love one another. The loving care that a church provides to those afflicted with dementia can have a profound impact on the greater community and allow them to recognize God's love at work.

As I write this, I am painfully aware that the needs of dementia patients may far exceed the church's ability to adequately help. Supplying sufficient assistance could easily deplete resources needed for other priorities. Nevertheless, I feel it is imperative for a local church to consider carefully the needs of those in their congregation who suffer from dementia. It is equally necessary for those involved in dementia care not to set overly high expectations for what the church can do.

Prayer

Heavenly Father, I am grateful that you have placed me in the body of Christ. I recognize that no local church is everything it should be, but because you are there, it has great potential. I pray for my church and other churches in my community, that you will use them to prepare your people to deal with dementia and then stand by families as they are called to go through the experience. I pray this for the good of all your people and for your honor. Amen.

12

Grow through the
Experience of Dementia

Those who experience the varied aspects of dementia grow as a result, and God is honored in the process. I am reminded of a saying attributed to Billy Graham: "Mountaintops are for views and inspiration, but fruit is grown in the valleys."[29] Growth in our character and relationships, both with others and with God, often occurs in the valley of dementia.

Five years after Dave was stricken, Denise got talking about how her life had changed though the course of Dave's decline. She said that had she known how difficult life would be, she would never in a thousand years have wanted to face dementia. Yet as she looked back, there were many things she was grateful for. She mentioned that she had learned to love Dave in a more unselfish way—more like God loves her. She had come to better understand the extent of God's love for her. She had learned to depend more on God for daily strength and emotional support. Her prayers had grown into cries to God for help rather than just telling God what she wanted. Denise went on to speak of how God was making her more patient and kind. Finally, she mentioned how meaningful her hope of heaven had become.

Just as Denise grew personally from her experience with dementia, so can everyone involved, whether patient, caregiver, or observer.

Prayer Life

Dementia, more than many other struggles in life, should teach us to pray. It will force us to depend on God and have daily fellowship with him. Our prayers will likely take on several of the following forms.

Lamenting

When we look at those we love and see the decline of their mind and the change in their personality, it is natural to respond with a sense of loss, grief, and even anger. Jesus himself experienced the loss of his relationship with his Father as we see in his lament, "My God, my God, why have you forsaken me?" (Matt. 27:46). We should never think we must always put on a good face when we pray, since God knows how we really feel. When dementia frustrates us, when we are angry with the victim, with the disease, or even with God, we should express it directly to him. Remember that dementia is foreign to God's originally good creation. It came as the result of sin. God wants us to lament and cry out to him in our frustration. When we do not feel God's presence, when we are not sure in our hearts that he really cares, we can let him know just how we feel. Honestly expressing ourselves is far better than turning our backs and running away from God. Even while we lament the tragedy of dementia, we can still trust that God is doing what is right. Note how the psalmist does both at the same time: "Trust in him at all times, O people; pour out your heart before him" (Ps. 62:8).

Requesting

God invites us to come to him as little children with our requests. Jesus told his followers to bring all of their requests to God:

Ask, and it will be given to you; seek, and you will find; knock, and it will be opened to you. For everyone who asks receives, and the one who seeks finds, and to the one who knocks it will be opened. Or which one of you, if his son asks him for bread, will give him a stone? Or if he asks for a fish, will give him a serpent? If you then, who are evil, know how to give good gifts to your children, how much more will your Father who is in heaven give good things to those who ask him! (Matt. 7:7–11)

The apostle Paul tells us: "Do not be anxious about anything, but in everything by prayer and supplication with thanksgiving let your requests be made known to God" (Phil. 4:6). Trusting that God, in his wisdom, has allowed dementia to cause our distress need not prevent us from asking him to grant us relief. A simple prayer such as, "Lord, Harry has been so upset today. I just don't feel I have the strength to truly love him and cope with this behavior. Please help me settle him down or else give me your strength. I don't care which, but please help." Pleading "I need you" is always appropriate. What should we ask God to accomplish through dementia?

- Pray that God will be honored.
- Pray for God to work in the spirit of the dementia patient, for peace and a consciousness of God's presence.
- Pray for spiritual growth in everyone involved.
- Pray for healing.
- Pray for unselfish love.
- Pray for wisdom and creativity to deal with each situation as it comes.
- Pray to see God working.
- Pray for a glimpse of God's love and faithfulness for which you can be thankful.
- Pray for the emotional, spiritual, and physical strength of the caregiver.
- Pray for other caregivers.

- Pray for those observing the loving care they see, that God would use this example to speak to them.
- Pray that when you ask for something specific that God will answer in the way he knows is best.

There is great consolation in knowing that we are not the only ones crying out for God to help us during our difficult days but that others are praying too. Most significantly, our Lord Jesus himself is praying for us: "Christ Jesus is . . . at the right hand of God . . . interceding for us" (Rom. 8:34); and "He is able to save to the uttermost those who draw near to God through him, since he always lives to make intercession for them" (Heb. 7:25).

Worship

Prayer is also an opportunity to pull away from our busyness and worship God as we focus on his greatness, love, and power—in other words, to worship. We also need at least a few moments each day to reflect on the character of our Savior while spending quiet moments remembering what he did for us on the cross.

Thanksgiving

It is not always easy to be thankful, yet the apostle Paul urged us to "give thanks in all circumstances; for this is the will of God in Christ Jesus for you" (1 Thess. 5:18). In another epistle he exhorted us to be "giving thanks always and for everything to God the Father in the name of our Lord Jesus Christ" (Eph. 5:20). Even when we struggle with adversity, we can find things to be thankful for if we try. Having a grateful heart not only pleases God, but it shapes our attitudes in positive ways. One key lesson learned from dementia for which we should be thankful is that it teaches us we are not in control but totally dependent on our Lord for his help. We should accept his daily help and presence with gratitude and tell him so in our prayers.

Love

Love is not purely unselfish. Our loving earthly relationships have some degree of selfishness associated with them. I certainly love my wife, Dorothy, but I acknowledge my love is somewhat selfish since her loving responses to me help me love her. Yet loving someone with dementia may be truly unselfish, which makes it similar to God's love for us, the purest form of love. He did not love us for what we could do for him. His love was totally undeserved and self-giving. A caregiver has an opportunity to practice that unselfish love. There is one significant difference between God's love for us and our love for one with dementia: God loved us when we were sinners living in open rebellion against him, while a victim of dementia suffers innocently. Knowing that should make loving those with dementia somewhat easier and more compassion-filled. Additionally, sufferers may have some appreciation of the love shown them and respond in loving ways themselves. Though at times unable to express it, deep in their souls they can appreciate and love their caregivers.

Trust

God does not expect us to understand all his reasons or methods. Moses gives us a good reminder of this: "The secret things belong to the LORD our God, but the things that are revealed belong to us and to our children forever" (Deut. 29:29). Recognizing our limitations, God declares: "For as the heavens are higher than the earth, so are my ways higher than your ways and my thoughts than your thoughts" (Isa. 55:9). Paul puts it this way: "Oh, the depth of the riches and wisdom and knowledge of God! How unsearchable are his judgments and how inscrutable his ways!" (Rom. 11:33). God knows we cannot fully comprehend him and his ways, but he wants us to trust him anyway. That is one of the greatest challenges of our lives. We need to have a big view of God that allows us to trust him when we do not understand and even when we are confused. Pastor Timothy

Keller quotes Evelyn Underhill, who insightfully writes, "If God is small enough to be understood, he wouldn't be big enough to be worshipped."[30]

When I think I understand a particular situation and therefore feel in control, I find it easy to trust myself and tend not to feel dependent on God. When dealing with dementia we very quickly learn that we are not in control, and, try though we may, we will never fully understand God's purpose in it this side of heaven. Dementia becomes a splendid opportunity to learn to trust God fully. As we go through the experience of dementia, the more we see God intervene, and the more our trust in him will increase. This can begin an upward spiral that will result in our ability to rely on him in increasingly challenging situations.

Most of us know of former slave ship captain John Newton, who after he was converted wrote the beloved hymn "Amazing Grace." Perhaps some don't know that he became a pastor. In a note to a parishioner serving as a caregiver he wrote:

> Your sister is much upon my mind. Her illness grieves me: were it in my power I would quickly remove it: the Lord can, and I hope will, when it has answered the end for which he sent it. . . . I wish you may be enabled to leave her, and yourself, and all your concerns, in his hands. He has a sovereign right to do with us as he pleases; and if we consider what we are, surely we shall confess we have no reason to complain: and to those who seek him, his sovereignty is exercised in a way of grace. All shall work together for good; everything is needful [necessary] that he sends, nothing can be needful [necessary] that he withholds.[31]

It may be easy for us to trust God when life is joyful and comfortable, but that is not the type of trust most honoring to him. A God-honoring trust grows when, struggling through difficulties, we cry in desperation, "God, I know you are there, and I trust you will do what is best."

Hope

When we start down the road of dementia, whether as patient or caregiver, our first response is not one of hope. We are looking at a tragic disease that profoundly changes all our lives and relationships, a condition for which medical science has very little to offer and that does not typically get better till death intervenes. What basis do we have for hope?

I do not claim there is an easy answer, but we find two helpful perspectives in the book of Romans. First, Paul teaches us that suffering coupled with the love of God, experienced through the Holy Spirit, initiates a cascade of events that moves from endurance to character building and in the end to hope:

> We rejoice in our sufferings, knowing that suffering produces endurance, and endurance produces character, and character produces hope, and hope does not put us to shame, because God's love has been poured into our hearts through the Holy Spirit who has been given to us. (Rom. 5:3–5)

This includes the suffering associated with dementia.

The second perspective comes from focusing on what Jesus endured for us: "What then shall we say to these things? If God is for us, who can be against us? He who did not spare his own Son but gave him up for us all, how will he not also with him graciously give us all things?" (Rom. 8:31–32). God has given us so much in Jesus that we can fully expect (hope) that he will carry us through our present trials.

But what is it that we hope for? If we are hoping for the dementia to be cured and for a return to a comfortable life on earth, we will likely be disappointed. Instead we should hope that God will accomplish his purpose through the dementia and that he will be honored. We also have hope for heaven; we anticipate the day when God will take all his children home to be with him, fully restored in the image of their Creator.

Finally, we are taught to look forward to a special reward

that will be given to those who endure through times of difficulty. James says, "Blessed is the man who remains steadfast under trial, for when he has stood the test he will receive the crown of life, which God has promised to those who love him" (James 1:12).

Yes! There are many ways that dementia can lead to growth in all those involved—patient, caregiver, and observer. As it does, God can certainly be honored and glorified. But there are specific ways in which patient, caregiver, church, and the larger community can all grow, and we now consider them individually.

Growth in the Victim of Dementia

I have seen the victims of dementia grow in specific ways. I will never forget my friend Bob, a careful and philosophic thinker. He always struggled with the idea that the gospel's free offer of salvation was so simple. He insisted that God must expect us to do our part to be saved. As dementia slowly began to take over his mind, he found that he could no longer keep doing all the good things he had done to try to earn God's pleasure. Finally, tears flowing down his cheeks, he told me he had realized that he could contribute nothing to achieve his salvation except trust in Jesus, who had done all that was necessary. I was dismayed at what Bob had to endure to come to this place of dependence and humility. But I appreciated that his dementia brought about some beneficial results.

We have spoken of the difference between our cognitive abilities and our emotional experiences. God is capable of meeting us on both levels. I have seen some highly intelligent people wrestle to simply trust God. Trust, though, is not just a cognitive activity; it also involves our emotions. We trust when we stop wrestling with our questions and rest in God. Jesus invited people to come to him as little children. Children may not cognitively understand everything, but they can emotionally trust. Early dementia may provide a renewed opportunity to trust and rest in God.

I have also seen some of my patients with dementia show significant growth in their overall spiritual lives. The Bible speaks of "the fruit of the spirit" (Gal. 5:22–23), which are character traits that God develops in us. Although far from a universal experience among those with dementia (and perhaps not even common), I have known belligerent people to become gentle and some impatient people to become patient through the illness. The Spirit of God was at work shaping their character. It is good if caregivers can recognize that God is working and do what they can to encourage this transformation. Their doing so is another way to honor God through dementia.

From a spiritual point of view, there is great value in being confronted by our weakness. Paul said, "For when I am weak, then I am strong" (2 Cor. 12:10). When we focus on all the things we can do and think how wonderful we are, it leaves little room for God. At times it takes dementia to humble us by allowing us to know how insufficient we truly are. Pastor Keller writes:

> Again and again in the Bible, God shows that he is going to get his salvation done through weakness, not strength, because Jesus will triumph through defeat, will win by losing, he will come down in order to go up. In the same way, we get God's saving power in our life only through the weakness of repentance and trust. And, so often, the grace of God grows more through our difficulties than our triumphs.[32]

Growth in the Caregiver

Those most likely to see spiritual growth are caregivers. They will grow as they pray, love, trust, and hope, and they may also experience the Holy Spirit's comfort and counsel more profoundly.

The Holy Spirit will also be active producing fruit in their character. Of all the fruit of the Spirit developed through caregiving, perhaps the chief one is patience. Likewise, caregiving promotes gentleness and self-discipline. Caring for someone with dementia also develops humility since the challenge of caregiving is so overwhelming. Caregivers quickly learn they cannot expect too much of themselves. Whether it is cleaning up a mess or realizing how much better the last meltdown could have been handled; it is a humbling experience.

Although not necessarily a deeply spiritual gift, rendering care teaches the ability to be creative and to improvise. There are no cookbook approaches to handling all the situations that arise when caring for a person with dementia. Thinking creatively can be a spiritual experience when it is done by listening to God's Spirit as he prompts us to think out of the box in new and fresh ways.

I need to mention one more trait caretakers develop—endurance. This becomes critical for the long haul. From visit to visit I have noted how caregivers increase in their ability to endure calmly as they face frustration day by day. I see them confirming the truth of Romans 5:3, which teaches that suffering nurtures endurance. On challenging days caregivers may feel that they are just stubbornly plugging away, but the fact is that their endurance is proof of their faithfulness. In the epilogue to Pastor Davis's account of his own dementia, his wife, Betty, shared the attitude that allowed them to endure. She wrote, "Live every day to the glory of God. Do every bit of good we can do for as long as we can do it. We have prepared for the worst and now we are going to live expecting the best. If the worst comes we are ready for it. If it doesn't, we will not have wasted today worrying about it. 'This is the day which the Lord hath made; we will rejoice and be glad in it' (Ps. 118:24)."[33]

Growth in the Church

There are several ways in which dementia can help a church congregation grow. First, it can give them the opportunity to serve unselfishly. Almost any church knows people with dementia and unmet needs, if not in their congregation, then in their neighborhood. Second, church leaders can help believers answer some of the theological questions that dementia raises. Some of these questions do not have easy answers, but they are worth asking, and providing answers a way to honor God.

Growth in the Community

Christians are observed by their non-Christian neighbors. They see when we reflect our Savior, and they know when we fail to do so. For many, the only picture they have of God or of Jesus is what they see in us. As the church demonstrates God's love to those with dementia, there may be some who come to appreciate God's love for them too.

Prayer

Heavenly Father, I am grateful for the way you take people who are unworthy of you, give them new life, and transform their character, preparing them for your eternal presence. It is heartening that you use dementia as a tool, whether in the lives of those with dementia, their caregivers, or others. Father, I submit myself to you to perform your perfect work and accomplish your honor and glory in my life. In your holy name I pray. Amen.

13

End-of-Life Issues

Dave's dementia progressed to the third stage, and he became totally dependent on Denise for care. He typically responded to her with a smile whenever Denise said, "I love you." But that was about it. With the help of a lifting device, she was able to get him up and into a wheelchair. She could no longer get him to use the toilet, and he was totally incontinent. He would sip liquids through a straw, but he had to be fed solids.

Finally their son, who had been visiting several times a week from across the state, had a serious talk with Denise. "Mom," he said, "what you are doing for Dad is getting too hard on you. It is time to make other arrangements." With some regret, she took his advice and looked for a nursing home that provided dementia care. I told her of my preferred facility, and by God's grace it was only ten minutes from their home. Denise immediately made arrangements for Dave to be admitted.

Once there, Dave was agitated, and Denise interpreted that as his being mad at her. For several weeks, he did not eat much in spite of the staff's faithfully trying to feed him. Hoping the staff would succeed in feeding him breakfast, Denise was there to feed him lunch and supper each day. In spite of that, he lost weight. One day I was there when she was feeding him and noted that he was having trouble swallowing and was choking on his food. I informed her that in the near future Dave was at high risk of aspiration pneumonia.

I also reminded her that I had promised to do everything I could to prolong Dave's life as long as doing so was appropriate. It was time for another discussion about that, so we arranged a meeting with Denise and other family members. After exchanging a few pleasantries I explained that Dave soon would develop pneumonia, and with his poor nutrition he would likely not survive it. It was time to write a "do not resuscitate" and "do not hospitalize" order, to which they agreed.

Less than a month later, Dave vomited one evening after eating and had a severe choking spell; the next day he developed a fever and became unresponsive. I was called and reinforced the order that no treatment was to be given since he showed no sign of distress. In two hours, with his family present, Denise holding his hand, and their son praying, the Lord took him home. It was very peaceful.

As we look at the final days of dementia patients, we are faced with a variety of questions. What is appropriate medical care? How do people with dementia tend to die? Is it ever appropriate to limit life-prolonging care, and if so, when and how? How can we promote comfort in the patient's last days? I want to share with you some of my ideas, but first we need to consider some biblical principles that underlie our response.[34]

Biblical Perspectives on the End of Life

Death Is Both Enemy and Defeated Enemy

Scripture gives us two seemingly conflicting ways to look at death. Our responsibility is to hold them in tension and decide which one applies to our specific situation. Paul says, "The last enemy to be destroyed is death" (1 Cor. 15:26). Even today death remains an enemy we must contend with. In his providence God has given us wonderful ways to combat death. Back in Genesis 1 God told us to "take dominion" (v. 26), and that led to all the medical technology we have at our disposal. God wants us to care well for the life he has given us, and part of that is to get medical help when we need it. We must, however, never put our confidence in medicine, for even when medical technology is used, it is God who heals. Therefore, if a patient with early dementia has a sudden cardiac arrest, we want to attempt resuscitation. If he develops an overwhelming pneumonia, we want to use a ventilator (breathing machine) for several days till antibiotics bring the pneumonia under control. These aggressive treatments are appropriate to fight the enemy of death when the chance of returning to a meaningful life is good.

Although death is an enemy, it's equally true that in Christ death has been defeated. Paul also writes, "'Death is swallowed up in victory. O death, where is your victory? O death, where is your sting?' . . . But thanks be to God, who gives us the victory through our Lord Jesus Christ" (1 Cor. 15:54–57). There comes a time when it is no longer necessary to fight death since it has already been conquered. At such times we can recognize death as a tool God uses to take us to himself. Ecclesiastes says, "There is . . . a time to die" (Eccles. 3:1–2), and the psalmist says, "Precious in the sight of the LORD is the death of his saints" (Ps. 116:15). That does not mean that God likes death—when standing at the tomb of Lazarus, knowing that he was going to raise his friend from the dead, Jesus wept (John 11:35). The challenge we face is deciding when it is appropriate to fight death by working with God to prolong a meaningful life and when we are potentially resisting him by merely prolonging a painful death.

The Timing of Our Death Is under God's Sovereign Control
God determined the length of our lives before we were born. He knows how, where, and when we will die. David could say:

> Your eyes saw my unformed substance;
> in your book were written, every one of them,
> the days that were formed for me,
> when as yet there was none of them. (Ps. 139:16)

Job echoes a similar thought:

> Since his days are determined,
>> and the number of his months is with you,
>> and you have appointed his limits that he cannot pass . . .
>> (Job 14:5)

While the length of our lives is determined by our sovereign God, at the same time, in ways that we may not fully understand, we have to make many choices that appear to affect how long we live. We need not be fatalistic, for in some way God's sovereignty works through our choices. Even knowing that, we are responsible for the choices we make.

Death Will Usher a Believer into God's Presence

Death for any believer, including those with dementia, is not the end. No! It is the beginning of a wonderful eternal life in the presence of God in heaven. This is such a critical perspective that we will return to it later.

Medical Decisions in the Course of Dementia

We must be careful not to confuse excellent medical care with the thinking that everything that can be done must be done, for, to be excellent, care must be tailored to each individual according to the medical context at the time. We must be constantly aware of and reevaluate the goals of care since our goals need to drive most of the medical decisions we make. These goals usually fall into three categories:

> Cure: Treating illness aggressively to prolong life as long as possible.
> Stabilize: Doing reasonable intervention to maintain a quality of life.
> Prepare: Planning for a good death with comfort and dignity.[35]

I have observed that those who come to the end of life well have been able to process and accept these goals. They gradually but purposefully go from a desire for cure to a choice for just comfort care as they prepare for death.

The aggressiveness of medical care should change as dementia progresses. In the early stages, when there may be some forgetfulness but life has many pleasures and meaningful activities, patients should receive the best life-sustaining medical care possible. If they develop pneumonia, they should likely be treated, even if it requires hospitalization and a short time on a ventilator. They should continue to have medical checkups to look for problems that will lead to more discomfort down the line, and these should be treated. If, for example, they are suffering from severe arthritis in their knees or hips, it is appropriate to have joint replacement surgery. If they are short of breath caused by a faulty valve leading to heart failure, they may consider valve replacement. At this stage of dementia the patient is likely to live another seven to ten years and should feel as well as possible during those years. On the other hand, it may be appropriate to stop doing cancer screening, since most cancers develop slowly and most patients will die of something else first.

Later in the course of dementia, as life expectancy shortens, pursuing certain aggressive treatments may no longer be appropriate. I recognize that mature Christians will think differently about end-of-life care, but speaking personally, if my life expectancy is two years, I do not want to spend a quarter of that time in rehab recovering from knee replacements. If I develop a cancer that would not be expected to kill me before I died of other causes, I would not want it treated. In the late stages of dementia there may be some potentially treatable but otherwise terminal conditions that I may not want treated, such as kidney failure. Frankly, I would rather not have dialysis. Let me die of kidney failure rather than severe dementia. In the event of such situations I would want legally executed documents ready at hand.

When my mother was in the final stage of dementia, we, her children, including my sister who had power of attorney, made clear that we wanted no treatment other than comfort care. We did not want her hospitalized or treated if she developed a severe infection that could rapidly take her life, such as pneumonia. On the other hand, if she developed a non–life-threatening but distressing infection that could be simply treated, such as a urinary tract infection, we did want her to receive antibiotics. The esteemed bioethicist Daniel Callahan wisely writes:

> I offer two principles. First, no one should be forced to live longer now in the advanced stages of Alzheimer's Disease than she would have in a pre-technological era. . . . With the severely demented patient, the rule should be: when in doubt, do not treat. Nothing good will be gained. Second, there is as great an obligation to prevent a lingering or painful death as to promote health and life.[36]

Hopefully by the time that patients lose the capacity to decide how they should be medically cared for, they will have an advance directive that names a surrogate who knows their wishes and informs the doctors. If they do not have an advance directive, it may be necessary to employ a lawyer to get a surrogate decision maker appointed. It can be challenging for a surrogate to make decisions in the context of dementia. In my experience many find it difficult to avoid either of the two extremes of pushing for overly aggressive medical care as death approaches or giving up too soon.

First is when the surrogate is unwilling to let the loved one go and has difficulty deciding to forgo or discontinue aggressive, often painful, and merely death-delaying treatments. I was sitting in a waiting room the other day next to a woman who, in the course of our conversation, found out that I was a geriatrician. Immediately she started to sob, telling me that her mother had recently died. In her sobs she blurted out, "And I insisted they keep her alive long beyond what she wanted. I was so selfish. I wasn't thinking of her but only about myself and how much her death made me hurt. I feel so guilty." It was hard to know how to react. I could only take her hand and tell her, "You did not make the choices that I would have made, but you loved her so much, and perhaps that is more important."

The other extreme is to underrate quality of life. Perceiving the patient's quality of life as unacceptable, the surrogate may forgo treatment that could be effective. Stephen Post speaks of a family who initially felt that life in a nursing home would make their father miserable but later concluded, "Dad really enjoyed the social interaction in the nursing home. We intellectuals are not a jury of Dad's peers."[37] In other words, the patient's quality of life as perceived by the patient may be far better than that perceived by loved ones or the medical establishment.

One question about treatment that comes up frequently is whether a feeding tube should be used to provide nutrition and hydration when patients are no longer capable of feeding themselves or of being successfully fed by others. The answer is a clear-cut no. It has been well proven in rigorous scientific studies that in the context of dementia, feeding tubes cause more problems than they prevent.[38] They neither prolong life nor provide comfort. Inserting feeding tubes, which is done by placing a small plastic tube through the wall of the abdomen into the stomach, while commonly done well, has the potential to cause serious complications. Tube feedings can cause diarrhea, which commonly leads to skin breakdown and bed sores. Feeding tubes seem to make sense if patients aspirate when swallowing, allowing food to get into the lungs. Yet feeding tubes do not prevent the aspiration of saliva into the lungs, and the presence of a feeding tube increases the risk of reflux of stomach contents into the lungs anyway. It is good to keep in mind that people in advanced stages of dementia stop eating because they are dying; they don't die because they stop eating. As death approaches and the body's systems begin to shut down, the stomach and intestines are no longer capable of accepting food. Forcing food at that point is useless since it is not absorbed and provides no nutritional benefit. Rather, it leaves one bloated and distended. A further complication of feeding tubes for dementia patients is that they can be distressing. To keep them from pulling on the tube, they often need to have their hands tied down or to be given strong sedatives, leading to further weakness and confusion.

Dying without the artificial hydration and nutrition that feeding tubes supply is not particularly uncomfortable. From the nutritional point of view, most people can live for more than a month without food, so rarely do patients die of starvation. If you talk to people who have fasted for long periods, they generally testify that the discomfort of hunger lasts only a few days. Also, without food, lactic acid will build up in a patient's body, serving as a natural sedative. We also must realize that dehydration is a natural part of dying. If fluid is forced on a weakened, dying heart, it typically goes to the lungs, which causes respiratory distress, or to the tissues, which causes uncomfortable swelling. Excess fluid produces discomfort and typically hastens death.

We also do well to realize how threatening, if not terrifying, aggressive medical care can be to one incapable of understanding the reason for it. People with dementia still feel pain, and even the pain of a needle stick can be disconcerting. Far worse is the horrendous fear of being taken away from the comfort of home and family and placed in a hospital room, especially an intensive care unit. There they will be confronted with a new set of faces every shift, awakened through the night for checks of vital signs, and subjected to all kinds of uncomfortable tests. It is no wonder most people who have dementia experience significant deterioration after a hospital stay. We need to think twice about the wisdom of hospitalization or even major outpatient tests before we commit to them. For those with advanced dementia, death may be a better alternative.

Over the years I have had many conversations with patients and their families about whether to pursue aggressive medical care at the end of life. Personally speaking, I want to receive every possible medical treatment when it is likely that I will be able to continue to serve others. However, when God no longer has work for me to do on earth, I do not want any life-prolonging care. At that point, I just want to be kept comfortable till God calls me home. One of my oft-used expressions is, "Heaven is so great that we don't have to fight to keep out."

Dementia Is a Terminal Disease

All forms of dementia progressively get worse; some such as early-onset Alzheimer's and frontotemporal degeneration cause deterioration faster than others. Dementia differs from other terminal conditions in that most of those with dementia worsen very slowly, and their life expectancy is difficult to predict. Nevertheless, all dementias are terminal diseases, and all victims will eventually die from them if another disease does not cause death first. Even if, by God's grace, medical science comes up with an effective cure for dementia, there will not be time to save the current generation of dementia sufferers. In view of that rather discouraging fact, dementia should be managed like any other terminal disease where comfort is more important than length of life.

How Do People with Dementia Tend to Die?

There is no stereotypical pattern to the death of those who survive long enough to reach the very end stages of dementing illnesses. One common theme is that poor nutrition compromises the immune system, making the diseased more susceptible to infections. Because they frequently aspirate food, saliva, or regurgitated stomach acid, the most common location of infection is in the lungs, typically pneumonia. Another common form of infection starts in the urinary tract and spreads to the blood—a condition called "sepsis." Either one of these infections can be treated with antibiotics, but that provides only a temporary solution at best since the problem is only going to happen again. Such a treatment

175

is more death-delaying than life-prolonging. When dying from these infections, the patient can almost always be kept comfortable with therapeutic doses of morphine or a sedative, without antibiotics or other aggressive treatment. I honestly cannot recall ever witnessing a dementia patient dying a very painful death. The gratifying aspect is that once death takes them to heaven, their suffering is over.

How Can We Promote Comfort in the Patient's Last Days?

At some point, as dementia progresses, all involved should accept that the goal of care becomes comfort rather than life prolongation. When this finally occurs, it is often wise to seek the help of a palliative care team or physician. Some communities have palliative care services for hospitalized patients only, but others offer them in outpatient clinics or even in the patient's home through a home health agency. These medical personnel, like their hospice counterparts, are experts at symptom control. Unlike hospice they are able to combine comfort care with aggressive treatment when applicable.

At such time as it is decided not to treat anything aggressively but offer comfort care only, it is wise to pursue hospice. Hospice organizations, now available across the country, provide expert professional care for those dying at home or, when necessary, in residential facilities, including nursing homes or hospitals. It is often mistakenly thought that hospice is simply to help people die well. That is not true. Hospices are interested in preserving quality of life till people die. This was well articulated by Dame Cicely Saunders, the British physician who founded the first hospice, who said: "You matter because you are you, and you matter to the end of your life. We will do all we can not only to help you die peacefully, but also to live until you die."[39]

When on hospice, the patient is seen regularly by a trained hospice nurse and as needed by chaplains, social workers, dietitians, and exercise coaches. Hospice will often provide home health aides for several hours a week to assist in such chores as bathing, dressing, and feeding. The programs are designed to slowly increase the level of support and frequency of visits till the patient dies and then provide grief counseling for loved ones afterward. Hospice organizations pay for all the medications related to the care of the terminal disease and provide equipment such as oxygen, hospital bed, or commode within the home. Personally, I find that some of the Medicare regulations regarding hospice are somewhat frustrating when dealing with dementia. Most onerous is the "six-month rule." To qualify for hospice the medical team has to certify that life expectancy is less than six months. Since dementia has such variable survival, it is frequently impossible to predict death six months in advance. There are many times when a person with dementia is fairly stable for some time and then rather suddenly deteriorates and dies within as little as a few days. That allows only a very brief time on hospice and fails to provide the patient its greatest benefits, which require time to establish. An additional frustration is that once on hospice, no further tests will be done. Generally, this rule is for the benefit of the patient, but it ignores the fact that some test results might suggest better ways to promote the patient's comfort.

The next thing that can be done to assure comfort at the end of life is to review all medical care and stop anything that does not contribute to immediate comfort. This is done routinely on admission to hospice, but it may be appropriate prior to that. It may no longer be necessary to treat elevated cholesterol. Life-preserving technologies such as implanted defibrillators should be turned off. Some restrictions can be relaxed. It may be all right to allow patients to enjoy some rich ice cream even if their cholesterol is high. A diabetic's blood sugar need not be treated aggressively or even monitored. Perhaps the insulin can be stopped, and they can enjoy an occasional candy bar or the cake that they have been deprived of for so long. They will probably feel better if they keep physically active, but long walks may be too much to handle.

Agitated patients may get worse as death approaches. Some of the really potent antianxiety drugs carry a warning of sudden death, which may prompt the medical team to refrain from using them. Whether these drugs truly increase the risk of dying is quite controversial; many experts and scientific studies argue that they do not. When someone is dying of advanced dementia and becomes agitated, it may be best to ignore those warnings, prescribe the medications, and take advantage of the relief they can provide. It is also likely time to stop the dementia drugs unless the patient clearly worsens without them.

Comfort care should always include prayer, though our prayers may take on a different form from earlier ones. Instead of praying for healing and continued life, we may start praying that the Lord would take our loved one home peacefully.

Another way in which I have seen end-of-life suffering limited is when loved ones, especially the caregiver, give the dying permission to stop fighting for life. Admittedly, those suffering the later stages of dementia may not understand what they are being told, but it is still worth hoping they will.

When our goal is to allow a dementia patient to die comfortably at home, a difficulty that can arise is the inability to control symptoms. Pain cannot be controlled; breathing becomes unacceptably labored; nausea and vomiting may be intractable. If, after doing everything possible at home, the victim is still in severe distress, it may be necessary to call 911 and have the patient transported to the hospital. If you do call for help, make sure you have the "do not resuscitate" document immediately available so the emergency personnel do not initiate lifesaving procedures. Like it or not, the hospital is sometimes the appropriate place for someone to die.

At times it is difficult to determine how quickly death will come. One of the advantages of being in hospice is that the nurses have the experience to make such predictions adeptly. When death seems imminent within twenty-four hours, it is time for the family to gather around the bed of the dying. They may be helped by quiet reminiscence and shared stories, savoring the good things of the past. It is good for loved ones to repeatedly assure the dying of their love and gratefulness for all the shared blessings over the years. Hopefully such a discussion has occurred long before, but if not, this may be the time to say, "Forgive me" or "I forgive you." It is also time for the family to express love for one another. Have quiet music playing and the TV turned off; consider singing together, reading the Scriptures, and praying. Commit the dying to the Lord and recognize that our Lord Jesus is there in this sacred moment. Remember, "Even though I walk through the valley of the shadow of death, I will fear no evil, for you are with me" (Ps. 23:4). Our Good Shepherd is himself at the deathbed.

What about Assisted Suicide and Euthanasia?

Physician-assisted suicide is now legal in several states, and there are initiatives in every state to legalize it. Euthanasia, while not legal in the United States, is allowed in certain countries in Europe and South America while being seriously considered in many others. Assisted suicide and euthanasia are often touted as a means of providing comfort and assuring a painless death. Many Christians faced with dementia, whether as patient or caregiver, will be tempted to pursue these options as they watch their relatively hopeless situation worsening. Those with dementia may fear losing control over their lives and want to free their families and caregivers from the burden of care. They might also understand that current laws require that the request for assisted suicide be made by individuals who know and understand what they are asking, and if they wait too long, they may not have the cognitive ability to fulfill those requirements. We need to be sympathetic toward those who desire assisted suicide, yet we must remind ourselves that all persons are made in the image of God and that God has put a divine stamp of protection over all human life. The principle we are given in Genesis 9 is clear: "For your lifeblood

I will require a reckoning: from every beast I will require it and from man. From his fellow man I will require a reckoning for the life of man. Whoever sheds the blood of man, by man shall his blood be shed, for God made man in his own image" (Gen. 9:5–6). Furthermore, the sixth commandment, "You shall not murder" (Ex. 20:13), surely applies here. As we mature in Christ we should desire to surrender more of the control of our lives to him while trusting him implicitly. Pursuing assisted suicide or euthanasia is just the opposite. It is saying, "I am not willing to trust God to do what is best. I alone know what is best for me, and I will do it." Such thinking runs counter to our faith.

The Final Destiny of Christians with Dementia

As we come to the end of our considerations on how God can be honored through the experience of dementia, we must think of the final destiny of those who have suffered from this devastating disease. In the case of a follower of Jesus, it is not what happens prior to death that is important but what happens after death. Meditate on the words of Scripture below until they lead you to worship our great God, who can use the tragedy of dementia to bring honor to himself.

Upon death all believers will go into God's presence:

> So we are always of good courage. We know that while we are at home in the body we are away from the Lord, for we walk by faith, not by sight. Yes, we are of good courage, and we would rather be away from the body and at home with the Lord. (2 Cor. 5:6–8)

> Let not your hearts be troubled. Believe in God; believe also in me. In my Father's house are many rooms. If it were not so, would I have told you that I go to prepare a place for you? And if I go and prepare a place for you, I will come again and will take you to myself, that where I am you may be also. (John 14:1–3)

There will be no more disease or death:

> He will wipe away every tear from their eyes, and death shall be no more, neither shall there be mourning, nor crying, nor pain anymore, for the former things have passed away. (Rev. 21:4)

Our bodies will be transformed:

> [He] will transform our lowly body to be like his glorious body, by the power that enables him even to subject all things to himself. (Phil. 3:21)

Our minds will be perfected:

> You have come to Mount Zion and to the city of the living God, the heavenly Jerusalem, and to innumerable angels in festal gathering, and to the assembly of the firstborn who are enrolled in heaven, and to God, the judge of all, and to the spirits of the righteous made perfect. (Heb. 12:22–23)

Suffering will be surpassed by glory:

> I consider that the sufferings of this present time are not worth comparing with the glory that is to be revealed to us. (Rom. 8:18)

As one body we will surround the throne of our Lord Jesus and give him the honor he so well deserves:

> They sang a new song, saying, "Worthy are you to take the scroll and to open its seals, for you were slain, and by your blood you ransomed people for God from every tribe and language and people and nation, and you have made them a kingdom and priests to our God, and they shall reign on the earth. (Rev. 5:9–10)

Within that vast throng will be many who have suffered the devastation of dementia while on earth. They will be standing fully

181

restored along with those who have selflessly cared for them. Now, at last, they will be able to truly honor God.

Prayer

Heavenly Father, I am thankful for your love and power and how you allow me to experience it. Lord, I see how dementia can be tragic, but at the same time I recognize that you are in control and that ultimately you will be victorious over all things, including dementia. Give me the faith to see your goodness; help me to experience dementia in such a way as to honor you. I pray this for my good and for your glory. Amen.

Acknowledgments

A book like this is never written single-handedly but is the result of many interactions and hard work on the part of many. I am deeply indebted to the many who have taught me much about dementia, both patients and caregivers. Many of them have illustrated how to experience dementia and honor God. My partners and staff in Zion, Illinois, have shown incredible patience with me and with the many we have served over the years. I am particularly indebted to Dr. Charles "Chick" Sell, who has been a constant encouragement. Chick and Lydia Brownback, the editor at Crossway, have been wonderful helps in turning "doctor talk" into meaningful writing. I have especially benefited from the careful review of the manuscript done by one of my previous partners, Dr. Lynnelle Flores. Advanced practice registered nurse (APRN) Mary Lewis, a dear sister in Christ in New Haven, has worked extensively with patients suffering from dementia at the Adler Center at Yale, and she provided wonderful advice and critique, as did Dr. Benjamin Mast. To each of these I am most grateful, and I know you will be too.

My parents, Bob and Lois, and mother-in-law, Edna Duenckel, each experienced dementia. They taught me some of the human aspects of this disease, and though now they are rejoicing with their Lord in heaven, I know they would be thrilled that their experience may be helpful to others and may bring glory to their Lord.

Dorothy has been my life's companion and encourager now

for forty-five years. To her I owe much. Dorothy means "gift of God," and indeed she is that to me. She too has made many contributions to the text.

I am grateful for the wisdom of the Scriptures, which I have sought to apply to the challenge of dementia. Most of all, I thank God for his love and how he has revealed it to me in the person of Jesus. "For from him and through him and to him are all things. To him be glory forever. Amen" (Rom. 11:36).

Appendix

A Letter to My Family

Dear Dorothy and any others involved in my future care,

As you know, I have given considerable thought during recent years to the subject of dementia. Though I am quite healthy now, I am aware that I may develop dementia in the future. If this should happen, I want to leave you with some guidelines for my care.

First, I want you to be totally free to apply these suggestions as seems prudent in the future. I am not attempting to lay down absolute rules. Furthermore, if you make decisions that you later believe were wrong, please know that I forgive you and do not want you to feel guilty about them.

In the early stages of dementia I hope that you will be patient with me, take time to know what I am capable of doing, and encourage me to do as much for myself and for others as possible. Feel free to let those directly impacted by my limitations know my diagnosis, but I prefer that it not be known by all my associates, since knowing I have dementia may significantly impact the way they relate to me. I will still want to feel that my life is meaningful, and in some way I would still like to help others. If I insist on doing things that may endanger me, please allow me to take some risks. If I am endangering others (perhaps driving beyond my abilities) be very firm about keeping me from doing so.

As my dementia progresses, I hope you will be willing to spend time with me, and even if you think I might not remember the time we have together, realize that I will have enjoyed the moment. Help me to stay connected with my past through stories and pictures. I hope you will make arrangements for me to hear the Bible being read as well as to hear old hymns I love. Talk to me about the Lord, his cross and resurrection. Speak often of heaven and what it will be like to enter God's presence. Give me some hugs to allow me to feel your love.

If I live into advanced dementia, continue to spend some time with me when you are able. Do not feel guilty if you decide I am best cared for outside the home. Dorothy, I want you to know how thankful I am for the ways God has gifted you to serve him. I want you to continue to do those things and do not want time spent with me to detract from your other callings. The same applies to all four of my children and each of my grandchildren.

As much as possible, keep me comfortable with medications but never initiate any treatment that would prolong my life. If I stop eating, I do not want artificial fluids or feedings; but keep offering to feed me. Do not treat infections unless it would contribute to my comfort. Please keep me out of the hospital if at all possible. I have always loved hospice and would be honored to be cared for by some of those great folk.

I know that being involved in the care of a dementia patient can be very difficult. If at the time I make it harder, please forgive me. I trust God will give you the grace to blame the dementia and not me. Know that I love you, and if I could, I would thank you over and over for your loving service to me.

I thank God that no matter what happens to my mind and body on earth, he will take me to be with him, and once there

I will look forward to being reunited with you, my dear wife, and with the rest of our family in the presence of Jesus with bodies and souls fully redeemed and restored in the image of God.

Love,
John

Notes

1. I am deeply indebted to John Kilner and his book *Dignity and Destiny: Mankind in the Image of God* (Grand Rapids, MI: Eerdmans, 2015) for this understanding of what it means to be made in the image of God.

2. Quoted in ibid., 97.

3. Joni Eareckson Tada, *The God I Love: A Lifetime of Walking With Jesus* (Grand Rapids, MI: Zondervan, 2003), 349.

4. Timothy Keller, *Walking with God through Pain and Suffering* (New York: Penguin, 2013), 89.

5. Note how Paul speaks of the image as being constant while what is being transformed is the amount of glory we are able to demonstrate. "And we all, with unveiled face, beholding the glory of the Lord, are being transformed into the same image from one degree of glory to another" (2 Cor. 3:18). Similarly: ". . . and have put on the new self, which is being renewed in knowledge after the image of its creator" (Col. 3:10). The image remains constant even while our knowledge is being renewed.

6. Robert Davis, *My Journey into Alzheimer's Disease: Helpful Insights for Family and Friends* (Carol Stream, IL: Tyndale, 1989), 131.

7. Alzheimer's Association, "10 Early Signs and Symptoms of Alzheimer's," accessed May 19, 2015, http://www.alz.org/alzheimers_disease_10_signs _of_alzheimers.asp#signs.

8. Celia F. Hybels, Dan G. Blazer, et al., "The Complex Association between Religious Activities and Functional Limitations in Older Adults," *Gerontologist* 52 (October 2012): 676–85.

9. Elisabeth Kübler-Ross, *On Death and Dying* (New York: MacMillan, 1969), chap. 2.

10. Davis, *My Journey into Alzheimer's Disease*, 47.

11. Ibid., 55.

12. "Thirty Percent of Caregivers Die," AgingCare website, accessed May 21, 2015, http://www.agingcare.com/Discussions/Thirty-Percent-of -Caregivers-Die-Before-The-People-They-Care-For-Do-97626.htm.

13. Kilner, *Dignity and Destiny*, 319.

14. Robertson McQuilkin, *A Promise Kept* (Wheaton, IL. Tyndale, 1998).
15. J. I. Packer, *God's Plans for You* (Wheaton, IL: Crossway, 2001), 154.
16. Jennifer Ghent-Fuller, *Thoughtful Dementia Care: Understanding the Dementia Experience* (CreateSpace Independent Publishing Platform, 2012), 169.
17. George Matheson, "O Love That Wilt Not Let Me Go," 1882.
18. Stephen Post, *The Moral Challenge of Alzheimer Disease* (Baltimore, MD: Johns Hopkins University Press, 1995), 3.
19. The Alzheimer's Association has a website titled "Singing for the Brain." There they state, "Singing is not only an enjoyable activity, it can also provide a way for people with dementia, along with their carers, to express themselves and socialize with others in a fun and supportive group. Hidden in the fun are activities which build on the well-known preserved memory for song and music in the brain. Even when many memories are hard to retrieve, music is especially easy to recall." Accessed December 23, 2015, https://www.alzheimers.org.uk/site/scripts/documents_info .php?documentID=760.
20. Rick Phelps and Gary Joseph LeBlanc, *While I Still Can: One Man's Journey through Early-Onset Alzheimer's Disease* (Bloomington, IN: Xlibris, 2012).
21. Stephen Sapp, "Hope: The Community Looks Forward," in *God Never Forgets: Faith, Hope, and Alzheimer's Disease*, ed. Donald K. McKim (Louisville, KY: Westminster, 1997), 94–95.
22. Benjamin T. Mast, *Second Forgetting: Remembering the Power of the Gospel during Alzheimer's Disease* (Grand Rapids, MI: Zondervan, 2014).
23. Phelps and LeBlanc, *While I Still Can*, 7.
24. Davis, *My Journey into Alzheimer's Disease*, 72.
25. Mast, *Second Forgetting*, 93.
26. These thoughts come from Benjamin Mast as quoted in an interview on the Desiring God website, accessed May 1, 2016, http://www.desiringgod .org/interviews/alzheimer-s-disease-the-brain-and-the-soul-an-interview -with-dr-benjamin-mast.
27. John Swinton, *Dementia: Living in the Memories of God* (Grand Rapids, MI: Eerdmans, 2012), 184.
28. Keller, *Walking with God through Pain and Suffering*, 268; emphasis original.
29. http://www.henrietsblog.com/2010/08/billy-graham-fruit-grows-in -valleys.html#.VXuET_lVhBc, accessed June 12, 2015.
30. Cited in Keller, *Walking with God through Pain and Suffering*, 255.
31. Cited in ibid., 266.
32. Ibid., 269.
33. Davis, *My Journey into Alzheimer's Disease*, 140.
34. I refer you to another book I wrote: *Finishing Well to the Glory of God* (Wheaton, IL: Crossway, 2011), which addresses these issues more fully.

35. These goals of care are nicely developed in a short book by Hank Dunn, *Hard Choices for Loving People* (Lansdowne, VA: A&A, 2001), 7–8.

36. Daniel Callahan, "The Elderly in Dementia," in *Dying in the Twenty-First Century: Toward a New Ethical Framework for the Art of Dying Well*, ed. Lydia Dugdale (Cambridge, MA: MIT Press, 2015), 183.

37. Post, *Moral Challenge of Alzheimer Disease*, 76.

38. S. Cai, P. L. Gozalo, et al., "Do Patients with Advanced Cognitive Impairment Admitted to Hospitals with Higher Rates of Feeding Tube Insertion Have Improved Survival?," *Journal Pain Symptom Manage* 45/3 (2013): 524–33; Elizabeth L. Sampson, Bridget Candy, and Louise Jones, "Enteral Tube Feeding for Older People with Advanced Dementia," *Cochrane Database of Systematic Reviews* 15/2 (2009), accessed October 11, 2016, http://onlinelibrary.wiley.com/doi/10.1002/14651858.CD0072 09.pub2/full; Thomas E. Finucane, Colleen Christmas, and Kathy Travis, "Tube Feeding in Patients with Advanced Dementia: A Review of the Evidence," *Journal of the American Medical Association* 282 (October 1999): 1,365–70.

39. Dame Cicely Saunders (1918–2005), cited in "Death, Suffering, and Euthanasia," College of Family Physicians of Canada website, accessed May 22, 2016, http://www.ncbi.nlm.nih.gov/pmc/articles/PMC2902937/.

Suggested Reading

Christian Perspectives on Dementia

Davis, Robert. *My Journey into Alzheimer's Disease: Helpful Insights for Family and Friends.* Wheaton, IL: Tyndale, 1989.

An insightful book written by a pastor and his wife during the early and mid-stages of his dementia. They give some feeling for what it is like to experience dementia.

Johnson, Richard. *How to Honor Your Aging Parents: Fundamental Principles of Caregiving.* Liguori, MO: Liguori, 1999.

A helpful look into the biblical basis for the relationship that should exist between adult children and their aging parents. Though not explicitly about dementia, it is largely applicable.

Keck, David. *Forgetting Whose We Are: Alzheimer's Disease and the Love of God.* Nashville: Abingdon Press, 1996.

Keck acknowledges the troubling theological questions that dementia confronts us with and presents some biblically grounded perspectives.

Kilner, John. *Dignity and Destiny: Humanity in the Image of God.* Grand Rapids, MI: Zondervan, 2015.

This theologian and bioethicist has rather exhaustively examined each of the biblical passages that relates to the image of

God and argues well that all humans are made in God's image, a fact that did not change at the fall.

Mast, Benjamin. *Second Forgetting: Remembering the Power of the Gospel during Alzheimer's Disease*. Grand Rapids, MI: Zondervan, 2014.

From among existing resources, this clinical psychologist and faculty member at the University of Louisville does perhaps the best job of combining a robust biblical theology with practical clinical experience in the care of those with dementia.

McKim, Donald K., ed. *God Never Forgets: Faith, Hope and Alzheimer's Disease*. Louisville: Westminster John Knox, 1997.

A series of essays emphasizing the hope available for those involved with dementia. Particularly helpful is the last chapter by Stephen Sapp.

McQuilkin, Robertson. *A Promise Kept*. Wheaton, IL: Tyndale, 1998.

The uplifting story of a love that matures through the course of dementia.

Sapp, Stephen. *When Alzheimer's Disease Strikes*. Palm Beach, FL: Desert Ministries, 2002.

A short book that looks particularly at the impact Alzheimer's disease has on others.

Swinton, John. *Dementia: Living in the Memories of God*. Grand Rapids, MI: Eerdmans, 2012.

A volume that provides a serious theological look at the issues of dementia, with helpful background reading to allow us to recognize some of God's purposes in dementia.

Secular Perspectives

Angelica, Jade. *Where Two Worlds Touch: A Spiritual Journey through Alzheimer's Disease*. Boston: Skinner House, 2014.

An estranged daughter comes home to care for her mother with Alzheimer's, and their relationship and love grow over the years.

Bell, Virginia, and David Troxel. *A Dignified Life: The Best Friends Approach to Alzheimer's Care*. Revised edition. Deerfield Beach, FL: Health Professionals Press, 2012.

The "Best Friends" approach to the care of persons with dementia is used in many treatment facilities across the country. It is based on the premise that the dignity of patients with dementia can and should be respected.

Coste, Joanne Koenig. *Learning to Speak Alzheimer's: A Groundbreaking Approach for Everyone Dealing with the Disease*. New York: Houghton Mifflin Harcourt, 2003.

Offers some very helpful suggestions on how to relate to what dementia patients say and how to treat them as full persons.

Genova, Lisa. *Still Alice*. Lincoln, NE: iUniverse, 2007.

A novel chronicling the experience of a brilliant professor entering and going through early-onset dementia. Released as a movie in 2015; well worth viewing.

Ghent-Fuller, Jennifer. *Thoughtful Dementia Care: Understanding the Dementia Experience*. CreateSpace Independent Publishing Platform, 2012.

A seasoned nurse in dementia care dissects how the various aspects of memory loss help us understand the world of dementia to more satisfactorily enter it and provide loving compassionate care. Packed with practical suggestions.

Kitwood, Tom. *Dementia Reconsidered: The Patient Comes First.* New York: McGraw-Hill, 1997.

One of the earlier books emphasizing the value of the victims of dementia as people and suggesting ways to preserve their dignity.

Mace, Nancy, and Peter Rabins. *The 36-Hour Day: A Family Guide to Caring for People Who Have Alzheimer Disease, Related Dementias, and Memory Loss in Later Life.* Baltimore, MD: Johns Hopkins University Press, 2011.

A classic text for caregivers; packed with practical tips.

Phelps, Rick, and Gary Joseph LeBlanc. *While I Still Can: One Man's Journey through Early-Onset Alzheimer's Disease.* Bloomington, IN: Xlibris, 2012.

A firsthand account of the challenges of dementia, with running commentary of ten years as a dementia caregiver for his own father. Many helpful perspectives.

Post, Stephen. *The Moral Challenge of Alzheimer Disease.* Baltimore, MD: Johns Hopkins University Press, 1995.

A thorough consideration of the moral challenges of Alzheimer's, including treating the victims as persons, diagnostic dilemmas, and end-of-life decisions.

Websites

Alzheimer's Association. http://www.alz.org.

A well-done website of the Alzheimer's Association. Includes a number of facts and figures along with articles and practical help.

Virginia Bell and David Troxel's "Best Friends Approach to Alzheimer's Care." http://bestfriendsapproach.com.

Explains the philosophy discussed in Bell and Troxel's *A Dignified Life: The Best Friends Approach to Alzheimer's Care*. Revised edition. Deerfield Beach, FL: Health Professions Press, 2012.

Resources about Suffering

There are many excellent books that discuss a biblical view of suffering. Three of my favorites are:

Carson, D. A. *How Long, O Lord?: Reflections on Suffering and Evil*. Grand Rapids, MI: Baker Academic, 2006.

A New Testament scholar discusses biblical perspectives on suffering.

Keller, Timothy. *Walking with God through Pain and Suffering*. New York: Penguin, 2013.

Biblically excellent and pastorally helpful.

Tada, Joni Eareckson, and Steve Estes. *When God Weeps: Why Our Sufferings Matter to the Almighty*. Grand Rapids, MI: Zondervan, 1997.

Joni, with Pastor Estes, relates Joni's tragic story, while developing a strongly biblical understanding of God's providence in our suffering.

Resources for a Christian Approach to the End of Life

Dunlop, John. *Finishing Well to the Glory of God: Strategies from a Christian Physician*. Wheaton, IL: Crossway, 2011.

Particularly relevant are the chapters that deal with suffering, the use of technology, and preparing for death.

Howard, Deborah. *Sunsets: Reflections for Life's Final Journey*. Wheaton, IL: Crossway, 2005.

A hospice nurse discusses and illustrates how we can come to the end of life with acceptance and peace.

Moll, Rob. *The Art of Dying: Living Fully into the Life to Come.* Downers Grove, IL: InterVarsity Press, 2010.

A journalist applies to the contemporary scene the ancient tradition of seeking a good death.

Verhey, Allen. *The Christian Art of Dying: Learning from Jesus.* Grand Rapids, MI: Eerdmans, 2011.

A theologian discusses what it means to die faithfully, drawing heavily on the ancient tradition of the Ars moriendi. He writes in the context of his own terminal illness.

General Index

Adam and Eve, 121; creation of, 105; fall of, 24
adult day-care programs, 91
advance directive, 49, 172
Alzheimer, Alois, 35
Alzheimer's Association, 89, 91; on information cards about dementia, 51; "Singing for the Brain" website of, 189n19; on ten early signs and symptoms of dementia, 44–45
Alzheimer's disease, 14, 34–35, 57; and the durability of emotional and procedural memories, 35; early-onset Alzheimer's disease, 35, 46, 175; factors that determine the impact of, 35; and life expectancy, 34; microscopic changes in the brain characteristic of, 35, 57; and a "possible" or "probable" diagnosis of, 46; three basic stages of, 34; treatment of, 57–58
anger: in caregivers, 79; in those with dementia, 73, 132
antidepressants, 58; citalopram (Celexa), 54, 58; mirtazapine, 56; sertraline (Zoloft), 54; trazadone, 56; tricyclic antidepressants, 56
anxiety, 31–32

assisted living facilities, 92; and Medicare, 92
atrial fibrillation, 36, 58–59; and vascular dementias, 59

benign senescent forgetfulness (BSF), 31, 43
blood thinners, 59; warfarin (Coumadin), 59
brain, the, 30; the aging of a healthy brain, 30–32; areas of normal brain function, 32; structural problems in (see brain tumors; normal pressure hydrocephalus; subdural hematomas)
brain injury, 15
brain tumors, 37
Buber, Martin, 104

Callahan, Daniel, 172
calling, 84; caregiving as a calling to love, 86–87; caregiving as a calling to serve, 84–86
caregivers, 18; and burnout, 90; challenges for, 71–72, 76 (see also dementia, behaviors of those with dementia); and depression, 79, 95; and fear, 79–80; and lack of support, 76; statistics on, 72, 77
caregivers, help for: assure that your own needs will be met,

Scripture Index

Also Available from John Dunlop

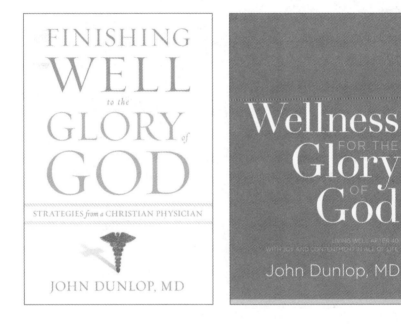

For more information, visit crossway.org.